Lighten UP

A HILARIOUS MEMOIR AND GUIDE TO REFLECTIVE MEDITATION

RODNEY LANEY

Post Hill
PRESS

A POST HILL PRESS BOOK
ISBN: 978-1-63758-010-3
ISBN (eBook): 978-1-63758-011-0

Lighten Up:
A Hilarious Memoir and Guide to Reflective Meditation
© 2021 by Rodney Laney
All Rights Reserved

Cover art by Cody Corcoran

Post Hill Press
New York • Nashville
posthillpress.com

Published in the United States of America
1 2 3 4 5 6 7 8 9 10

In loving remembrance of
Aunt Mern, Aunt Lucy, and Robert Miller.

Contents

Introduction 9

The Dam Breaks 16

How I Discovered Meditation 17

My "Movie" Begins 22

Momay...26

The Towers...32

Mrs. McNeil...37

Mrs. Offenberg 39

Mrs. Mary...41

Uncle Kenny 50

Mrs. Gatlin 53

The Key 62

The Fellas..73

The Holy Ghost...82

Paper 86

Luther 93

Hoop Dreams 96

Peanut 99

Boy Scouts 107

The Dirty South...................................112

Noodle 121

Blindsided 124

Straight Street......................................127

An Odd Year 133

Frankly Speaking..................................137

Stuck...140

Donkey Kong..149

Hot Dogs 153

Medication 164

Mr. Miller 167

Man Up 174

Eastern Christian..................................176

Tomas 180

Broken Codes..182

The Slicing..186

Dougie Fresh 194

Crab..201

Michelle 205

Rebellion...207

Mr. Sherman 209

Cheeba 212

Sherice 217

"We Need a Plan" 224

The Oak Tree 229

Party Time 232

The Fall(s) 234

Defender 238

The Question 251

The Big Move 252

My "Movie" Ends 253

The Meditation 255

Epilogue 269

Acknowledgments 271

About the Author 272

Introduction

Truth be told, I never wanted to be a comedian. I tried it out of curiosity and then, fortunately, discovered I was good at it. But since I started reviewing my life through reflective meditation, I came to understand that my love for comedy came from something that happened when I was in the fourth grade.

My mom had moved from South Carolina to Paterson, New Jersey when she was eighteen years old and gave birth to me two years later. My dad was in the photo album, but he was never in the picture. With only an eighth-grade education, my mom hustled between factory jobs, which provided us some stability but kept her busy.

I wasn't the best student, but in the fourth grade, I was selected to participate in a math bee, which is similar to a spelling bee but with math problems. I was excited and told my mom about the contest, hoping that she would attend. She said she would try. On the day of the competition, the other students and I assembled backstage and were given numbers and final instructions before being seated on the stage. The curtain opened, revealing an auditorium full of moms and dads. I fidgeted in my seat as my stomach turned over. I just wanted to lose and be done with it. When they called my name, my legs felt like tree stumps. I managed to walk to the center of the stage, only half paying attention to the panel while looking for my mom in the audience. The lights glared, making it hard to see faces in the audience. They gave me a multiplication problem. I calculated for a second, spoke the number that popped into my head, and heard a round of applause.

I returned to my seat, relieved and elated. I continued searching for my mom. After a few more rounds, only one other student and I were left. He answered incorrectly, and if I got the next problem right, I'd win. A member of the panel monitored the time, and when she raised her hand, it meant you were out of time and the competition. I had drawn a blank on my problem. Blinded by the lights, I stood on the stage, simply staring at the audience. The monitor's hand started rising, along with my anxiety. I blurted out, "172." A wave of cheers rushed the stage. I had won. As I received the trophy, I could see that my mom wasn't there. Although she was missing, the other people there gave me something that at the time I didn't understand.

Fast-forward ten years. I was in the Air Force stationed at Wright Patterson Air Force Base in Dayton, Ohio. I'd been invited by a fellow airman to do an open mic at the local comedy club, which I had forgotten about. And that was a good thing since I probably would've chickened out. The guy who'd invited me did five minutes to utter silence. You would have thought the crowd was meditating. Nervous, with no idea what I was going to say, I walked onstage. My personality cracked them open, and the few stock jokes I told worked. I reveled in their joy. Afterward, I rode back to the base with the other comic…in dead silence.

I wish I could say that's when my comedy career started, but it didn't. Once I got to Barksdale Air Force Base in Louisiana, I tried comedy again. The outcome was different this time. I bombed in front of my fellow airmen and friends. I felt as if I had been dropped out of a B-52 bomber. I was just awful, so I gave up.

After my service, I worked in the laboratory at Hackensack University Medical Center, but something was missing. The job never gave me that feeling I'd had onstage. So I just had to try stand-up again. After a number of successes, I got booked to do a popular radio show in New York City. It was the first time I'd heard my name on the radio. I rode the momentum, and my career began to blossom as I made appearances on Comedy Central, *The Late Late Show*, and HBO.

Although my comedy was considered clean, some of my jokes demonstrated an unhealthy sentiment that arguably stalled my career. Thanks to meditating, I've come to realize that some of my jokes came from a deeply unconscious resentment toward women stemming from my childhood—no surprise there. But that was only one of the many discoveries I made about myself and how my sub-conscious behavior confined my potential and even restricted my relationships.

There are tons of bitter comedians. I believe it's because we spend so much time trying to make other people laugh that we forget sometimes to make ourselves laugh. We get caught up trying to *make it* while witnessing other comics' progress, and too often, resentment seeps into our consciousness. Thanks to the method of meditation I learned, I know that will never happen to me.

I discovered this meditation in 2013. It taught me how to uncover all the cardinal memories that had been weighing me down and how to discard them. With the clearing came clarity and an openness that made it possible to laugh hardily at other comedians.

I had two key realizations, although both sound trite. The first was that I was looking for validation through performing, and the second was that true validation doesn't come from the stage; it comes from within. I'd read books and understood concepts intellectually, but I'd never seen any real change before I learned to meditate. Meditation allowed me to experience those realizations in my subconscious and make a real transformation. Once that weight was lifted, I was truly able to lighten up—hence this book's title.

Now, my mission is to promote awareness of this reflective meditation so people can free themselves from their subconscious memories that are linked to fear and anger, the root causes of suffering, anxiety, and depression. I know that once people are freed from these negative emotions, they will lighten up and fulfill their highest potential.

How cool would it be to watch a person go from being a self-centered NYC-based comedian unable to achieve true joy and prosperity to an egoless meditator who lives in a state of harmony, grace, and abundance? Now imagine if you could see the transformation while laughing out loud in the process. You will. That's the bold promise I'm making.

By reading about my meditative process, you'll see how I liberated myself from the *remembered life* and came upon true freedom. Seeing how I achieved it, you'll have the opportunity to do the same…if you want to and are willing to learn the process.

If you don't want to suffer or see others suffer, then I hope to convince you to start doing reflective meditation sooner than I did. I put off meditation for years. I had trust issues. It took me a while to stop meditating with my back to the wall with one eye open.

Where I'm from, being still with closed eyes meant you were on P-dope (aka heroin).

My comedy career has spanned more than two decades. I went from telling jokes in the best holes in the wall in North Jersey and hawking comedy tickets in Times Square for stage time to booking television appearances in Holland and England and returning to entertain my fellow military members in Kuwait, Oman, and Saudi Arabia.

Even though I studied books by the sages J. Krishnamurti, Eckhart Tolle, Sri Nisargadatta Maharaj, and Ramana Maharshi, all of which reference meditation, I never actually meditated. It was one of those things I would "get around to." All that changed when I discovered this unique meditation in an unpremeditated way. I was hooked immediately and began spending three to six hours a day meditating. It was just that powerful. I invested more time in meditation than in any other endeavor in my life, including stand-up.

You might be able to get a doctorate in theology, but it doesn't mean you're enlightened. Spirituality is not exactly quantifiable. Or is it? The measures I used to understand my growth were the clarity of my thinking and how long my mind stayed brooding on an event that triggered a spiral of negative thoughts and emotions. As a result of my introversion, I could replay an event in my head endlessly. After I began meditating, those same triggers lasted only minutes or seconds, and sometimes they didn't even register.

Due to my dedication and rise in consciousness, the meditation center I participated in invited me to events reserved for senior meditators. I was even asked to guide other members. Traveling the country performing stand-up offered an unexpected benefit: I could also visit the various meditation centers throughout the world. And although the method was consistent, each guide's tutelage gave me different perspectives, which gave me a more comprehensive understanding of the technique, making my education unique and exceptional.

This book is a memoir, but it's more than that too. It's a testimonial for meditation told with a humorous narrative uncommon to most spiritual texts. You'll join me at the point when I found meditation. Then we'll travel back to my childhood in Paterson, New Jersey, where you'll see how the person least likely to become enlightened surmounted suffering, and you'll learn about all the impediments that could've constrained my spiritual growth and true prosperity. The final part of the book is a quick step-by-step guide to the techniques that have helped me. And you'll be able to find more tips at www.RodneyLaney.com.

BUSINESSES CAN BENEFIT

The media talks about the lack of diversity and inclusion in businesses. Proponents of diversity say that an honest dialogue needs to take place between employees and business leaders. But what happens after the dialogue? What happens after the conversation that possibly offended and hurt your employees or peers? Are they supposed to pretend that the conversation hasn't been seared into their memories? You can label the meeting a "judgment-free zone" all you want, but it's simply unrealistic to think that people will engage in a real conversation without holding on to what is said or heard. You have to address the issue at the time of emotional crisis.

A solution to this issue comes from my mom's old demand: "Sit your butt down and be still and think about what you did." Her advice is more relevant today than ever. The only thing missing from her timeless advice is "and then what?" What are you supposed to do with the analysis? This book answers those questions, which can help business leaders in their conversations about diversity. The meditation given at the end of this book is perfect for those difficult conversations. I'd even argue it is indispensable.

YOU CAN BENEFIT

In this book, you will learn about meditation techniques and why reflective meditation is one of the most powerful tools available for your spiritual transformation. If you practice this form of meditation, it's likely you will experience many benefits, such as being able to rest in stillness longer and forgive completely. You will be emotionally lighter since the thoughts that are anchored by negative emotions will disappear. Even your face may physically change and brighten up as you discard the years of baggage. You will be able to see people as their true selves and not through your shrouded perspective.

So, whether you're interested in this for yourself or your business or workplace, let's lighten up.

The Dam Breaks

As I sat in a small room in a legless chair, a tear formed. Its formation was magnified by the stillness. It swelled in the corner of my closed eye, then rolled down my cheek and fell in silence. It carried decades of mental conditioning. Something deep inside me broke, and a rush of ecstasy washed over me, drawing me into a living emptiness that was unknowable yet infinitely real. It could be expressed only by my stream of tears.

I was experiencing a breakthrough in meditation and undergoing a glimpse of what I would call the supreme perspective. As I was set free from my personal mindset—the mindset chiefly responsible for anxiety, suffering, and unhappiness—my world changed in a way that is beyond my capacity to explain. I can only describe it here.

How I Discovered Meditation

I split open the piece of "chicken" to investigate its realness. It damn sure tasted like yard bird. I'd heard that Veggie Heaven's tofu was unbelievable; I had to agree. The Asian waitress topped off my water, left a fortune cookie with the pink check, and disappeared behind the galley doors before I could ask for a doggie bag. I cracked the cookie and quickly read the fortune, which promised that "big changes" were coming. The only change I could see coming was from my last twenty-dollar bill.

I stared into my phone's blank calendar as if doing so would make a stand-up gig appear. June of 2013 was dryer than British humor. I had nothing significant on the books until the fall. The cashier gave me a cursory smile, then put three quarters in my palm, making me second-guess my decision to stop eating meat. The tofu was tasty, but it wasn't cheap.

My sweet tooth drew me to the cake showcase. My eyes ping-ponged between the red velvet, the carrot cake, and my wallet. Eventually, they settled on something heavenly: a meditation brochure sitting next to the dessert display. Now that was smart marketing.

I scanned the leaflet judiciously because I had been interested in meditation since I started reading spiritual texts. The language in the pamphlet had enough familiarity to be meaningful and enough novelty to be intriguing. According to the brochure, a ten-minute introductory lesson was free on Tuesdays. I said, "What the hell," then called and set up an appointment.

The next Tuesday, when I disturbed the tiny bells hanging on the back of the meditation center's door, they returned the favor. For unknown reasons, jingling bells always unsettled me. A meditative melody played while a variety of mountainscape images illuminated a TV monitor. A shoeless white guy opened one of three doors off a narrow hallway and eased the door shut behind him. He introduced himself as John and offered me tea and coffee in a peaceful New Agey tone. He asked me to take off my sneakers; I assumed because he was five foot four and didn't want to look up at me. I tried to recall if my socks had holes in them. I have a long toe that has a wicked habit of gnawing through socks. But it was too late, so I kicked off my shoes into an array of footwear, hoping for the best, then followed John into the Universe room, a room holier than my socks.

Standing at a whiteboard, he began the lesson.

"The reason we do this meditation is to change humans from being incomplete to complete..."

When I listen intently, my brow furrows. I lose myself in talks and rarely give a nod or an utterance that ensures I'm following. This can be disconcerting to speakers, which is probably why John asked, "You follow?"

I nodded. He motioned to seven magnetic rings, each bigger one encircling the smaller ones in varying colors, each representing a level of enlightenment.

"The more you empty your mind, the more you enlighten to truth, and the less burdens you will have. And eventually, you'll reach a level of no mind," he said.

After the introduction, John approached me and sat uncomfortably close. "How wonderful would it be to live in a world where you could walk up to strangers, sit down, and join them to eat?" he asked.

Great, since I'm on a budget, I thought.

"That would be cool," I said.

Then the biggest Korean I'd ever seen filled the entire doorway—or escape route, depending on one's perspective. He stuck out his long arm for a handshake.

"I'm C-Bon," he said.

"I'm Rodney."

"Follow me," C-Bon said.

My fight-or-flight response was eased by his childlike smile and warm voice. He ushered me into a smaller room at the back of the center. I assumed he was the "closer." There he asked what I thought about the meditation. It resonated with me more than I had anticipated, I admitted. I had come with two intentions: to listen and to avoid drinking any Kool-Aid. *'Cause that's how they get you!*

"My brudda, you sign up tonight," C-Bon said.

His voice didn't go up at the end of his sentence, so what should've been a question sounded like a statement. His six-foot-six, three-hundred-pound solid physique made it a demand. Rarely, if ever, do I decide on anything contractual on the spot, but my interest had been piqued, and I didn't have an excuse not to sign up. Not that I wanted one. Plus, I had a fail-safe: As I'm a comic, if something bizarre were to happen, at the very least, I would get a joke out of it. Obviously, I was hoping for something greater—much, much greater.

I decided to sign up that night mainly due to my gut feeling. C-Bon extended his arm again to give me a congratulatory handshake. I didn't want to give him my credit card info because automatic payments, without automatic deposits, equals automatic stress. Coincidentally, I had enough cash to avoid the plastic.

"When can you start, my brudda?" C-Bon asked.

"June first."

I usually start new endeavors like a kid in a bouncy castle. I hop in with zeal and keep going until my motivation deflates, but this time would be different, I hoped. The volunteers, known as helpers, promised that if I meditated diligently, I would reach a state of "no mind" relatively quickly. My initial goal was to "enlighten" as fast as possible. Every day I hurried to the center to do nothing. Actually, that's not true, but from the outside looking in, that's how it appeared.

Each session started in the Universe room with a brief lecture by helper C-Bon. He restated the purpose of the meditation and the ultimate purpose of human existence. Then the "throwing away" of my "life lived" would commence. I was instructed to bring up all my childhood memories and use the center's method to discard them.

The chairs were legless; they provided enough support for my back but not enough for my tush. I needed extra pillows and extra gym time for squats. In the beginning, my discomfort was distracting. My mind did all it could to derail my progress. But after the first week, I was able to sit longer as my booty and the rest of my body interfered less with the stillness.

I spent hours reviewing different aspects of my entire life categorized by theme: family, money, enemies, relationships, work, school, places lived, fortune and fame, health, and things I wanted to do. The more memories I discarded, the more memories surfaced—memories that I buried or thought I had forgotten. The more I reviewed, the faster I could discard, to the point that each memory lasted as an image for only a millisecond. By June's end, I'd meditated an incredible ninety-six hours.

Although I was instructed to refrain from staying in the memories, some would suck me in, especially the ones I hadn't thought of in years. It felt rude to not even acknowledge them. It would have been like having an old friend whom you haven't seen in years stop by your house, and you slam the door in their face, saying: "You should've called first."

With the reflective meditation, I was reviewing a "movie" costarring my family and friends, set in all the places I'd been. A movie that was written and directed by and starring Rodney Laney. But there was one major problem with the movie.

My "Movie" Begins

The principal action in this type of meditation is discarding—meaning throwing away the thoughts and images that arise, and even the body and the universe. I use the term "discarded" at the end of each chapter to represent that step.

The italicized text gives context to the story and isn't necessarily part of my recall during the meditation session being described.

I'd learned to avoid the La-Z-Boy chair because even the best meditators could be heard snoring in it after the lights were dimmed. And whereas others sat in the legless chairs, I preferred a regular chair when one was available. An old knee injury prevented me from that guru-ish Lotus position. Unlike most meditators, I wore socks, not for my benefit but for theirs. After we said a prayer of gratitude in Korean and in English, I closed my eyes and began discarding.

My grandmother died after giving birth to her fourteenth child. There are questions regarding her death since she didn't die in the hospital but at home. My grandfather was killed years later, a subject rarely

discussed. Mom feared her father because he was a harsh disciplinarian. She buried with her dad the fear of any man.

Mom's attitude was the reason she went to New Jersey. Her younger sister, Mildred, moved to Paterson after a pregnancy and shotgun wedding. Aunt Mildred's sisters-in-law began bullying her, so she called Mom, who arrived at their doorstep yelling, "Come outside."

Two years after Mom arrived at their home, I arrived at hers.

In my meditation at the center that day, these are some of the thoughts and images that came up.

A cylinder block crashed through a windshield, cracking the glass and shattering my sleep. I sat up and listened. I kicked off my Spider-Man comforter, then tiptoed toward the screaming—Mom's screaming.

Howard, my stepdad, backed away from his knife-wielding wife. Mom stalked him around his Gran Torino, stopping to smash a side-view mirror, baiting him to come after her. When that didn't work, she scraped the door with her knife. Green paint chips fell onto the broken glass. Through the screen door of our balcony, I saw Mom's puffy eyes, consumed by her fury, but she didn't see me.

Discarded.

Our house was standoffish. The two-family home, owned by Uncle Kenny, Mom's brother-in-law, sat deeper on its lot than the neighboring houses. Other houses on North Fourth Street had a backyard, but ours had only a front yard, making it recede and look as if it didn't want to be bothered. Mom prohibited me from leaving the yard, preferring that I play closer to the house, away from the sidewalk and all the fun.

During my preschool summer, I used my Big Wheel and Tonka truck in our yard as lures for neighboring kids. No one took the bait. Then one day, I saw Elroy, a slim, shades-wearing teenager who sported a mini Afro and Dr. J Converses. He lived a couple of houses over, but I had never met him. I knew his name only from overhearing it in the neighborhood. He lounged on the shaded steps of the boarded-up house adjacent to ours. Even on this stuffy day, he looked cool. After noticing me, he motioned for me to come over. But he was on the other side of the fence. Elroy waved again as if he had something to tell me. I stepped onto the sidewalk, leaving the gate behind me open, and sat next to Elroy.

Next to our house on the opposite side of the abandoned house lived a white family with three boys and a dog. Their dog barked at me as if I had bones in my pockets. Until Elroy, that dog had been my only source of attention when I was playing in the yard. Elroy perked up as the youngest brother from that other house approached. Before he reached us, Elroy said: "Punch him in the face." *What?* I thought. But said, "OK."

When the kid got close enough, I followed orders, popping the kid in his fleshy jaw. Then I nonchalantly returned to my perch next to Elroy. The kid scurried through his gate and raced up his steps. Behind him, the door slammed shut, sounding like the blast of a shotgun.

Elroy's laughter was as reassuring as his pat on the back. His approving eyes hid behind his sunglasses until he snatched them off. I turned to see what captured his attention. It was the three brothers tramping toward us. The eldest, who was Elroy's age, led the rush, followed by the middle brother with the assaulted one in tow. I looked for Elroy, but he'd vanished. The door of the condemned house swung shut. I stood in front of the abandoned building alone.

"Who punched you in the face?" said the eldest.

A long, pale finger pointed at my nose.

"Well, punch him back in the face."

The boy zealously carried out his orders, cracking me on the chin. Void of instruction, I stood there blankly. With instant justice rendered, they left. Their retreat prompted a wide-eyed peek from behind the dilapidated door. Elroy stepped into daylight while surveying the area for the brothers. He approached.

"Why didn't you run?"

"Because you didn't tell me to."

Discarded.

Mom stood over me as I crouched in fear, or anguish, or perhaps anger while frantically trying to tie my shoes. Again and again, the knot failed, and with each failure came a scolding and then a lashing.

Discarded.

Momay

How do you ask a blind person to watch your five-year-old child? "Do you mind look…I just need you to watch…take care of my son," my mom said to Momay, a woman I didn't know and who couldn't see.

The curious flicker of lightning bugs was overshadowed by the taillights of my uncle Gucci's car. He reversed the car down the driveway and onto the main road, scraping the car's front end on the curb and blazing up the road. Momay stood next to me as I watched my uncle and mom speed away into the hazy twilight.

While their trip to Lancaster, South Carolina, had ended, mine was just beginning. They were headed back to New Jersey, while I had been left behind with a strange woman—a strange blind woman whom I didn't know and, in all honesty, didn't care to know. Momay, a family friend, was giving Mom the break she needed. A deep sigh ended the long farewell. I continued watching them drive up the road until they were out of sight.

Lancaster's quiet gave volume to my thoughts, which were filled with cuss words. Since my voice didn't matter—given that my protests about coming here had been ignored—I resolved not to use it. But I would quickly discover how far-sighted it was to remain quiet around Momay.

The situation offered me a new freedom and took one away. I could make all the funny faces I wanted without getting backhanded for it, but I had to learn the whole "ma'am/sir" thing, or else I would get pinched.

"You want something to eat, baby?"

"Yes."

"Yes what?"

"Yes ma'am."

The city's landscape I knew was now far away, both physically and mentally. Concrete and caution had become dirt and boredom; squeaking intercoms and dinging elevators had become chirping crickets and cooing woods. A thick loneliness wafted through Momay's home. That and the smell of mothballs. The blinds dissected the sunlight, creating a pattern of alternating light and dark streaks across the old country-folk furniture. The doors creaked. They were tattletales and snitches, who would've never survived the streets of Paterson had they been human. Always ratting to Momay about my whereabouts.

Whenever Momay said, "It's time for bed," I wondered: *How does she know?* What was her clue that it was time to send me into that dimly lit chamber? I thought about lying, saying, "It's still daylight outside," but I couldn't risk getting pinched. Nothing smarts like a grandma's pinch, not that she was my grandma. The smell of cigarette ashes and butts had seeped into the guest room's comforter. There wasn't a mirror, only bare gray walls.

A gentle raspiness colored Momay's voice. The softness made misunderstandings common, especially if she wasn't angled in my direction.

"I said bring me my shoes, not screws."

"I said ice, not knife." *Thank God.*

One thing she made clear: I wasn't allowed in *the back*.

Her small brick home sat above a main road facing a gas station; a car would pass by every one or two hours. The highlight of my day was watching people pump their gas, something New Jerseyans weren't allowed to do. Her front yard sloped steeply, and one misstep could lead to my tumbling into an orange clay ditch.

Momay didn't mind my reticence and never pressured me to talk. For the first few days, we kept to ourselves on the porch in a blind, dumb silence. She stared off into nothingness while I snuck peeks at her, wondering if she had Daredevil's superpowers. But I doubted it when I found an eye booger in my eye. No adult woman would ever let that go unnoticed. She would either make you stick out your tongue and use your saliva to clean your face or, even worse, would lick her own thumb and wash your face with her spit. If the boogers in my eyes didn't get dislodged when Momay wiped my face in the morning, they were part of my ensemble for the rest of the day.

The brown sap on the bark of the only tree in Momay's yard begged for attention. One day I stuck a twig into the icky fluid. Although it smelled sweet, I thought better of tasting it, certain it was poison. My afternoons had been lapsing at the same pace of the drippage and seemingly with the same purpose: waiting to slowly drop out of sight. Then something rustled through the forbidden stalks, grabbing my attention. Was it a man or an animal? I dropped the twig, ready to dash inside the house. Whatever it was finally left, but not before arousing my curiosity.

Before the screen door smacked shut, Momay warned me: "Be careful, and don't go in the back."

What was in the freakin' back? I had learned that adults loved "the back." Where's everybody? "Out back" or "around back."

Whenever I headed to the rear, I got stopped short and had to "back up." If Momay did have a superpower, it was telecommunication. If I was even looking out the back door, before I could form the thought, she appeared to say, "Don't even think about it."

I knew how deeply Momay slept based on how far her wig slid to one side. If I could see her ear, she was napping. But if I could see the stocking cap, she was down for the count. One day, gauging by her hairpiece, I had at least a half-hour to explore. I snuck out using the front door since it was the one least likely to snitch.

A dirt path led into a thicket, then bent left until it vanished into a maze of tough weeds. I knelt at the clearing, tied my shoes tightly, then looked over my shoulder, ensuring that Momay wasn't at the screen door ready to flip her wig.

Weeds covered in gray-green moss squished when I poked them, releasing a pungent smell of corn and rain. How they remained moist in that Carolina heat puzzled me. Clusters of yellow jingle bell-shaped flowers marked the entrance to the woods behind Momay's house. Crackling bugs warned their gang members that fresh meat was coming. The dry grass crunched under each step as I made my way deeper into the jungle. The insect chatter gave way to distant voices and dogs barking. I stood still, gripped by the thought *What if Momay wakes up early?* If she did, she would surely be calling. And if I didn't answer, she would know where I had gone and would pinch the bejesus out of me. But I needed only a few more steps to see the back. I crept forward, peering through the brush, and saw two men near caged dogs. The barking beefed up as if they knew I was nearby. The men looked in my direction. I squatted out of sight. I'd seen enough. It was time to head back to the front.

I hauled boogie toward the house. Only a few yards separated me from the entrance when I heard the bushes rustle. Something parted the stalks. An animal. *Probably rabid.* Was it coming from behind or from my side? It was circling, stalking, ready to attack. It lunged from the grassy underground. I couldn't run. I couldn't scream. I couldn't think. I could only see the snake.

The viper sidewinded to a halt, seemingly locking eyes on me. Its forked tongue darted from its scaly face, tasting my fear. It stood its ground, poised, while I was completely rattled.

Before it could strike, two men charged from the bush with shovels and hoes, then began chopping through its rubbery flesh, hacking at it ferociously. Flecks of snakeskin flew over their heads, and blood pooled at their feet. I covered my eyes, feeling my way through the bush until I reached the grove's opening, where I could see Momay on the porch staring with her unseeing eyes

"Baby?"

I went to her side. She draped a warm arm over my shoulder, pulling me, suspending me in the safety of her embrace.

For the first couple of weeks, a car pulling in the driveway would spark me to run to the door, hoping to see the emerald Chevrolet with Mom behind the wheel. But the letdowns got old. So when a car stood idling in the driveway one day after I'd been there a few weeks, it was an intrusion on my and Momay's time.

Momay turned off the heat under her pots in the kitchen, then wiped her hands on her cooking towel in a way that suggested she wasn't surprised by the visit. I sauntered behind her. In the driveway sat the green hatchback, where I had hoped it would've been at least a dozen times before.

I ambled through the side door toward the precious smile and blissful bosom of my mother. I was going home.

The gravel crunched under the tires as we pulled out into the street. Memories of Momay flashed through my mind as she stood on her porch, waving farewell. I could see her smile. She must've been using her superpowers.

Discarded.

The Towers

Howard was a short, dark man with an Afro. For most of the time I knew him, I don't think I ever saw him smile, at least not at me, not even after my return from Momay's house, but that all changed a few weeks later when my big-bellied mom left for the hospital.

"What would you like me to have?" Mom asked.

"A sister," I said.

Natasha fulfilled my wish, becoming the adored addition to our family. Howard especially adored her.

Natasha's presence didn't stop the fighting. Fed up, Mom decided to escape from her husband, leaving him with only a fork, a knife, and a pot. So she thought. Unfortunately, she also left a leather jacket by Aunt Doris, her sister-in-law's house, which had a receipt for the deposit in the jacket with the new address. Aunt Doris believed that families should be together. So she forked over the receipt to Howard, her brother-in-law—who, to Mom's chagrin, found us quickly enough to almost help unload the moving truck. Howard pleaded for another chance while holding his daughter in his arms.

We had moved to building one of the Riverview Towers, four sixteen-story buildings located along the Passaic River in New Jersey. Our two-bedroom apartment, 14C, had four rooms plus a bathroom. "Tasha" slept in her crib in the room with Mom and Howard, giving me my own room.

One day, on the ground floor of a green warehouse called Public School 28, I stood in front of Mrs. Degroat's classroom. I don't remember what I did to get in trouble, but it didn't take much with Mrs. Degroat. My stern and stubby first-grade teacher studied the palm of my hand like a heroin addict looking for an injection spot. I hadn't made many friends, so being in front of the class at least got me noticed. Mrs. Degroat raised her handmade ruler-paddle, then whacked my paw with precision. She eased back in her chair, enjoying the rush. My attempt at shaking the stinging away failed.

The 2:30 bell enlivened the classroom. Books were closed and chalkboards erased while kids lined up backpack to gut, ready to bolt at the 2:35 sound of freedom. I wasn't part of the frenzy. At 2:40, I hit the playground and lay inside the concrete tunnel, which resembled a giant anus. I hung out there until hunger moved me.

During her first few years at the Nabisco factory, Mom worked swing shifts. When she worked the second shift, I was left in Howard's care. After school, I'd knock on the door, push the bell, then knock again, making sure I didn't knock too hard "or else." When it opened, he would stand inside, bare-chested in khakis, scolding me without saying a word.

Mom left me with hearty hot meals before leaving for work. Unbeknownst to her, I had stopped asking for seconds since it was never permitted.

"You had enough," Howard would say.

Once home, I was prevented from going outside for three reasons. First, in order to go out, I had to ask Howard. Second, he would've had to respond. Third, I knew I would get that look. I overcame Mrs. Degroat's ruler, but Howard's look cut deeper than any lashing.

With no chance for seconds or dessert, I took solace on the balcony since going there didn't require his permission. On some level, I was outside. The balcony was more than an amenity; it was my pie in the sky. Our terrace hung fourteen stories high over West Broadway, a street lined with a hodgepodge of businesses: Chinese restaurants, barbershops, and hole-in-the-wall bars.

My uncle Gucci loved a good hole in the wall. Out of Mom's six brothers, he was her closest. Whenever he was around, cigarette butts, beer bottles, and decks of cards accented the kitchen and the balcony. The only drawback to his visits was that he would take over my refuge. I wasn't allowed on the porch while the adults were doing their thang. Only after Uncle Gucci and Mom finished their smokes did the balcony become mine again.

The railing came up to my chest, but I could've easily hopped over it if I'd wanted to go splat. I shook the four-foot-high steel mesh banister daily to check its sturdiness. A bird landing on the railing would stir jealousy. I wanted to soar, if only for a few seconds. The pigeons would give me the side-eye from the ledge as if they could hear my thoughts.

A ruffled banner partitioned the balcony into two sides, ours and the neighbors'. It wasn't the late-night wails that made our neighbors in 14B mysterious. That wasn't a big deal on a floor with sixteen apartments. It was the hollering plus the rare sightings of them that made them odd. They were never seen in the hallways, the elevator, or the incinerator room. It was as if they didn't want to be seen, only heard. All that changed one day when *she* looked at me over the banner.

She was my age, had my complexion, and my, my, my.

"Hi," I said.

"You talk to yourself often?" she asked.

"What? I wasn't talking to myself."

"Your lips were moving."

She dipped out of sight and then reappeared, seated at the opening of the partition closest to the building. I rearranged the patio furniture and slid between a table and chair so I could get closer.

"What's your name?" I asked.

"Stacey."

From then on, Stacey and I met on the balcony. From then on, I chomped down my food and didn't think about seconds.

Once the school bell rang, I was first to line up. I ran home with a jangling book bag, papers flying, leaving a paper trail, all in hopes of talking to Stacey—the half of her face I could see, anyway. Sometimes I waited for her against the wall, but she didn't come out. That made each time she did more precious. I began wanting to see both eyes, both ears, and a full smile.

Then one night, something unbelievable happened.

It was not a dream. The rumbling in the living room made it certain. I sat up in my bed, knowing that the screams I heard were real. I scuttled down the hallway into the kitchen, wearing my onesie pajamas. Mom's face was buried in her palms. Howard was peering over the balcony railing, and alongside him, puffing a cigarette, was Uncle Gucci. I heard sirens, saw whirling lights, and heard "Oh my God" wails from the other balconies. I inched toward the open patio door. I had just raised a foot to cross the threshold when Uncle Gucci saw me.

"Uh-uhm! You can't come out here. This is something you don't want to see," he said. He turned me around and then ushered me back inside the kitchen.

35

Mom took my hand and led me back to bed.

"What happened?" I asked.

Another scream snatched our attention toward the front door. Chatter from walkie-talkies echoed in the hallway. Someone banged on the door of 14B. Mom stuck me in the bed and turned out the lights, leaving me alone with one thought. *Did something happen to Stacey?* I tiptoed toward the door and cracked it open, listening. Mom's voice cracked as she said, "I can't believe she committed suicide."

The following day, I laid the news on my classmate, Dave Beason. "The lady next door committed suicide," I said, wondering if the word "suicide" baffled him like it did me. "Why she kill herself?" Dave asked. Damn. He was smarter than me.

"Stacey's mom jumped from our balcony, landing on a gate below, splitting her body in half."

"You're lying."

"I ain't lying."

I wished I were. I only told Dave, but the news raced throughout the school. After repeatedly being questioned about it, I started shrugging my shoulders and keeping silent.

After delaying the inevitable, I slid out of the giant concrete anus after school with stomach pangs. When I got to our building, the numbers on the elevator flickered. I was hoping the day would be different. That Stacey would be on our balcony, and I could say something to her, possibly spark a smile on even a quarter of her face. Unfortunately, I would never see her again.

Discarded.

Mrs. McNeil

Nothing drove home new vocabulary for me like an emotional outburst. It was how I learned most of my new words. I remember the day I learned what "paramedic" meant.

"Hey, what was it that Mrs. Brown suffered from?"

"Hysteria."

"What about Ms. Jenkins?"

"Delirium."

"And Mrs. Cartwright?"

"A nervous breakdown."

Many of the words were seared into our memory as teachers were carted off screaming foul language.

"What's a bastard?" someone asked Mrs. McNeil, my second-grade teacher. She tilted her head to the side, thinking of an adequate response as she viewed a classroom full of them. "That's when a child is born without their parents...um...being married."

After a second, it registered. *Well, that means...* I didn't know if it was a good thing or a bad thing, only that it was my thing. It sounded badass, like "son of a bitch." Bastard Laney. I asked other kids to see who qualified for this exclusive club. Turns out the club wasn't that exclusive.

"Can only kids be bastards?" I asked Mrs. McNeil.

She smiled coyly. "No, sometimes an ex-husband qualifies."

Drilling and hammering echoed in the hallway as construction workers labored on the school's roof that spring of second grade. The heat from the unusually sweltering spring day made the classroom a slow cooker. Each tick of the clock's second hand was punctuated by the blow of a hammer. The days were the type that made you want to shout, which is exactly what someone did one day. Mrs. McNeil leaped from her seat and ordered us to remain in ours. Some students listened; some didn't. Mrs. McNeil ran into the hallway. My uncle Gucci's previous warning, "This is something you don't want to see," kept me in my seat.

"Get some ice!" someone yelled.

Curiosity overwhelmed me. I joined the huddle at the doorway. A student ran down the hall with an empty bucket. Mrs. Teneal, our teacher's close friend, was slumped against the wall, holding her bloodied hand in agony. The student returned with ice in the bucket, and something was placed in it. The ambulance guys took Mrs. Teneal away. One of them carried the bucket with her little finger. "Eww, that's nasty," a student cried out.

Mrs. McNeil turned toward us. "Get back in the classroom."

She would earn the nickname "Ms. Pinkie" after the tragedy. Kids are cruel.

"What will those ambulance guys do with her finger, Mrs. McNeil?"

"They are not called 'ambulance guys,'" she said.

Discarded.

Mrs. Offenberg

The only teacher who didn't paddle me was Mrs. Offenberg, but that wasn't the only reason why she was odd. Her oral lessons grossed me out. They were not about history but about how to properly brush our teeth. *How did the fanaticism begin?* I wondered. Had she caught a whiff of a student's breath and thought, "Good God. I've got to fix this!"

On a cardboard poster, she created a calendar grid with our names and spaces to check off and chart the tooth brushing. I imagined she thought, *War on crime? Nonsense. War on gingivitis!* She intended to clean up the hood one mouth at a time and improve the air quality to boot.

Daily, Mrs. Offenberg guarded the classroom door armed with her chart. She stopped each of us for tooth inspection as if we were cattle.

"Open up," she ordered me one day. She stuck her nose inside my mouth and tooled around. "Did you brush your teeth?"

I tried to answer. "Yaaaaaaaaa."

"Are you sure? It doesn't look like it."

"Yaaaaaaaaaa ahh ushh ay eeeth!"

I could taste her skepticism. I wanted to bite her nose off like the animal I was being treated like. I imagined her running down the hallway, noseless and screaming, "Where's that ice bucket?"

And other teachers asking, "Why was her nose in his mouth?"
Ms. Pinkie would be joined by Ms. Nosey.
Discarded.

Mrs. Mary

The fourteenth floor of our apartment building smelled of bacon in the mornings and cornbread in the evenings. The smells came from 14D, where Mrs. Mary lived. The door fanned her cooking down the hallway from the steady stream of kids coming and going from her apartment. Mom worked swing shifts at the Nabisco factory, as I mentioned, so whenever Howard's shift changed and he couldn't watch us, Tasha and I had to go to 14D.

A black mole hung over her lip. An old scarf squeezed the jumbo rollers in her hair. She wore a grandma's nightgown and open-toed hard-bottomed house shoes that were weapons of ass destruction. Tasha hated going to Mrs. Mary's; for me, it was the lesser of two evils.

In 14D, the living room was full of brown toddlers and kids from building one, splayed over the carpet facing a floor-model Zenith. It took balance to wade through the minefield of brats on route to go potty. One misstep and you would smash a rascal's pudgy finger or baby toe.

My sister and I were regulars at Mrs. Mary's. The kids who I thought were fortunate were the ones who went only once or twice a week, a privilege not afforded to the regulars. There were other privileges, such as answering the door, going into the kitchen, or sitting on the sofa. Only Mrs. Mary's descendants were allowed at the kitchen table or in the back.

Each kid carved out a spot on the shaggy green carpet. I would sit in one spot for hours and never complain about my ass bone cutting through my butt cheeks. I couldn't jeopardize my prime spot, which had a clear view of the Zenith. While others watched television lying on their stomach, I sat cross-legged with my back straight. Proud. I knew the end table was the boundary. If anyone sat on the other side of it, they were subject to scolding and banished to the back by the fish tank. A scolding would ruin my plans for the sofa.

One day, two newcomers arrived. Where were they going to sit? The first immigrant stepped onto the carpet in his buttoned-up shirt, thin glasses, and shiesty smile. He probably went to private school. He stood tall, speaking with Mrs. Mary like an adult. The nerve. Then the edges of Mrs. Mary's lips curled, revealing her teeth. She actually smiled. My spot on the sofa was in jeopardy.

The glasses of the second newcomer, a girl, were unapologetically thick. Until then, the only person who had worn glasses thicker than mine was Mr. Magoo. This was my kind of girl. I figured she had to be at least seven or eight—same age as me. She scanned the room for a seat, looking to sit down without the fanfare of....

"Vincent, say hi to everyone. Everyone say hi to Vincent," Mrs. Mary said.

I mumbled the greeting and scooted closer to the wall, making room for....

"Everyone say hi to Mietta."

Mietta nestled into the space I had cleared for her. Mrs. Mary went into the kitchen. I listened for the fridge to open. Then the cabinets. And, alas, the cans. She was starting dinner, giving me the time I needed. I whispered to Mietta, "Which floor do you live on?"

"Four. You?"

"I live next door. You know Antonio? He lives in 4G."

"Maybe. What's he look like?"

"Short, pea-headed, always laughing."

"Kinda cute?"

"I don't think so. Never mind."

"Pea-headed—that's all the boys in building one."

I ran my fingers through my hair, certain it was nappy. As we sat there, the doorbell rang three or four times an hour. Our heads would turn to see who was being freed. With each departure, more space on the floor became available. The clearing allowed me to spread out and watch *Three's Company* comfortably. Jack Tripper wanted to know if the lady in the episode was dating. He needed to be subtle in how he approached the question. I knew then what I was supposed to do. I had to be subtle.

"Do you have a boyfriend?" I asked.

I didn't know what "subtle" meant.

"Uh-uh."

Mrs. Mary plopped down in her post. "Maleek, turn to channel seven," she said.

Hart to Hart, one of Mrs. Mary's favorite shows, came on. The star was a self-made millionaire whose determination got him what he wanted. That's exactly what I was going to do. I was going to get what I wanted.

In class, I studied the students, looking for someone to help me with my dilemma. I needed a nerd. My friends and I thought Dawn Blakely had gunpowder in her armpits, the way her hand shot up to answer questions. I figured she had to know.

"How does somebody make a girl their girlfriend?" I asked her.

"You can't make someone anything," Dawn replied and reinserted her nose in her book. I sucked my tooth at the future feminist and kept scanning the room. The girls swooned over a man-size third-grader named Anthony Robinson. I waited until recess to get his advice so he wouldn't tease me in front of the class.

At recess, a girl named Jocelyn tap-danced over the ropes, pattering on the blacktop while two other kids, Aicha and Duane, turned the two ropes for double Dutch. Anthony Robinson's fingers clutched the fence he was facing; he resembled an inmate contemplating escape.

"Looking for your beanstalk, Maskutchi?" I said.

"You looking for a garden to plant your pinto bean head?" Anthony said.

"Good one, good one. "

"Don't get me started on those goggles."

"Chill, chill. I gotta ask you something."

"I ain't do it."

"You probably did."

He leaned back against the fence. Two girls, Dawn and Diane, hung from the monkey bars, their skirts whirling in the wind.

"How did you get Sharon to be your girlfriend?"

Anthony smirked while looking around the playground to figure out which girl I was trying to get. I braced myself for the ridicule.

"Just make a note," he said.

"A note?"

"Yeah. Put two boxes: one for no and one for yes."

"That's it?"

"Worked for me."

Later that day, I knocked on Mrs. Mary's door, and lo and behold, Vincent opened the door. Mr. Bullwinkle had already earned the privilege to answer the door? I pushed past him looking to see if my soon-to-be girlfriend had arrived. She had. I had the note tucked away in my backpack. All bookbags were kept in the corner, so I had to fish out the note before putting my bag away. I checked all the compartments. *Oh no*, I thought.

The search attracted Mrs. Mary's gaze. "You lose something, Rodney?"

I shook my head no, then took my seat. Jasmine, Mrs. Mary's granddaughter, sat at the head of the dining room table drawing and tossing balled-up sheets of paper without regard for where or on whom they landed. Mrs. Mary's princess was immune to punishment. She randomly fired cheap shots. "Rodney, why your glasses so big?" she asked me.

Retaliation toward the beloved tattletale was a no-no, so I usually ignored her, but that day I couldn't; Jasmine had something I needed.

I waited for Mrs. Mary to leave the sofa. She was eating her prunes, so it wouldn't be long before she'd have to get up to go to the bathroom. We were under her intense surveillance because of Maleek. Gum was forbidden, and Mrs. Mary eyed us vigilantly for sticky candy ever since Maleek had ruined a section of her carpet. A wad of gum had fallen out of his mouth while he slept. After Mrs. Mary cut the gum out of the rug, she yanked down Maleek's pants and tore...his...ass...up. No more candy for me. Maleek lived in constant anxiety after that.

When Mrs. Mary stood, our necks snapped toward her. We exhaled when she headed to the bathroom. It was her poop time. I peeped at Jasmine while she scribbled on her notepad with multiple pencils lying on the table. Watching her wasn't going to get me what I needed.

"Jasmine, can I borrow a sheet of paper and pencil?"

Ridicule was coming; I just knew it. Jasmine ripped out a leaf and slid her red pencil to the edge of the table, then returned to her drawing. It was so easy that it felt like a setup. I snatched the paper and pencil before she changed her mind and returned to my spot. I looked over my shoulder and saw that Jasmine's head stayed down. I drew the boxes first and then, in my best penmanship, wrote, "Would you like to be my girlfriend?"

I slipped the note to Mietta. While she chewed over my proposal, I chewed on my fingernails. Mrs. Mary's abrupt return meant the prunes had worked. She probed the room with her X-ray vision. I used spasmodic eye movement to signal to Mietta to hide the note. She slid the note into her pants. I felt Mrs. Mary's gaze on the nape of my neck.

"Pssst," Mietta called and mimed her words. I jerked my head toward Mrs. Mary, cuing Mietta to keep quiet. Mrs. Mary didn't spank little girls, but the boys received no mercy. Mietta's mimicry confused me.

"What you two doing over there?" Mrs. Mary asked.

"Huh? Nothing," I said.

The balcony door opened. If Mrs. Mary ended up asking for my note, I had a clear path to the porch for a nosedive. Breezing in from the balcony came my bushy-mustachioed savior, Mr. Jim—Mrs. Mary's husband. Nothing bad happened in Mr. Jim's presence. He rarely came out of their bedroom. He was rugged and weird, which is why I liked him. One time he even let me see his gun.

"Don't let the missus know I showed it to ya," Mr. Jim said.

I nodded.

"It shoots tiny people," Mr. Jim said.

"Like midgets?"

"No, tiny pebbles."

Thank God he wasn't shooting little people. He was shooting squirrels. No one said anything about Mr. Jim's strange game, but I suspected it wasn't legal. He would skin them in the bedroom, and Mrs. Mary would make squirrel stew. These were the people entrusted with my well-being. Once Mr. Jim threw a squirrel hide on Jade, Jasmine's older sister, and I learned the meaning of "conniption."

On this day, Mr. Jim, a fanatic for westerns, tickled Jasmine and then placed the *TV Guide* in front of her. She put her paper aside, opened the guide, and started her daily errand. When Jasmine wasn't around, he gave me the honor of circling all the westerns in the *TV Guide* in red pencil.

"What's for dinner?" Mr. Jim asked.

Mrs. Mary stood. Maleek flinched. And I turned to Mietta.

"What is it?" I said.

"I need the pencil," Mietta said.

I slipped it to her. She marked a box, then folded the paper right as Jasmine shouted, "I need my red pencil, Rodney."

Why was she so damn loud? I sensed Jasmine's gaze as she pushed away from the table. Mietta slipped me the pencil—which became a dagger, a dagger that I considered plunging into Jasmine's bony butt, the butt that was in my face, the face that smiled and handed her the red pencil.

Was all this worth what was in Mietta's pants? The doorbell rang. Vincent started to rise, but Jasmine's stiff-arm gesture stopped him, and she opened the door. "There's a police officer here," Jasmine said. Every head in 14D whipped around toward the door. Police? I thought Mr. Jim was going to jail for squirrel homicide.

Mrs. Mary came out of the bathroom. "Mietta, get your stuff," she said.

Was she under arrest? Was my future girlfriend a criminal? As Mietta gathered her stuff, she saw the questions swirling in my eyes.

"My mom," she said.

"Oh, cool."

I noticed her mother's gun and decided that I could wait for my answer to the note. While her mom arrested everyone's attention, Mietta stuck the note in my hand. After she left and after Mrs. Mary settled into the sofa, I unfolded the note.

"What you smiling at, Rodney?" Jasmine said.

Mind yo business, Jasmine.

Fast-forward to another day. ABC's Friday-night lineup had started. All of the kids were gone except Tasha, Mietta, and myself. My girlfriend rarely stayed late. Maybe her mom had shot someone. My girlfriend's mom carried a real gun, one that didn't shoot pebbles.

Mrs. Mary's rollers flattened against the arm of the sofa. Drool seeped from the corner of her mouth as air gurgled from her throat. Mr. Jim's snoring reached the living room from their bedroom. Tasha was asleep too. How Tasha could sleep through the racket boggled me.

"It's an old-fart competition," I said.

Mietta laughed out loud, then covered her mouth. We laughed in silence. I scooted closer to her and put my arm around her waist. She scooted next to me. It was like prime-time TV. We were Hart to Hart on the Love Boat headed to Fantasy Island.

I came up with a fantasy that didn't require Tattoo or Mr. Roarke. I eased over to my bookbag, scribbled a note, then slid it to Mietta. She read it and rolled onto her side. Her pupils filled the frames of her glasses. So sexy. Was I serious? She flattened the note, put an X in a box, then handed it back.

"Really?" I said. Mietta nodded. I thought for a minute. "Where?" Mietta shrugged her shoulders. *We'll need a romantic place*, I thought.

"How about the staircase?" I said.

"OK."

It was set.

I lay in my bed, elated that I was going to "do it" to Mietta. There was only one issue. What the hell did "doing it" mean? I had all weekend to figure it out.

I sailed straight to 14D on that glorious Monday afternoon. I didn't know much more about "doing it." I figured if we both took our pants off, we should be able to figure it out. Even if Vincent answered the door, it wouldn't matter. I was about to *do it*. I arrived before Mietta and secured our spot on the carpet. I needed a plan that would get us in the hallway together. Maybe if I was allowed to answer the door, I could sneak us out.

I craned my head every time the doorbell rang. Mietta had missed the *ABC Afterschool Special* and *Diff'rent Strokes*. My excitement waned during *Good Times*, and my curiosity was piqued during *What's Happening!!* She didn't come that day or the next. When Matthew sat in her spot, I asked Jasmine: "What happened to Mietta?"

"Her mother found another sitter for her, I guess."

I sprawled over the floor—no more *Happy Days*.

No matter how many newbies arrived or how cluttered the carpet became, I always took up two spaces. Just in case.

Discarded.

Uncle Kenny

Kenny Simmons, a garbage man, married Doris, who gave him seven kids. Doris introduced Mom to Howard, Doris's brother-in-law, making us part of the Simmons family. So I thought. Uncle Kenny fathered eight kids (that we knew about): Dee Dee, Tammy, Rocky, Kennedy, Kim, Tootsie, Tara, and Shannon, whose mom wasn't Aunt Doris.

I bit Tootsie once or twice when I was four. I don't remember why, but Aunt Doris never forgot it. Whenever I visited, she would always ask: "Are you hungry, Rodney?" As if that were the reason I had bitten him. It wasn't my fault he tasted like steak. Rocky, the eldest, teased me for biting and said something I never forgot: "Only cowards bite."

The Simmons were the Black Brady Bunch plus one. The only differences were that they all had the same father and there wasn't a maid. But Uncle Kenny cleaned house in his own way. In their backyard, he made a craps table out of an old pool table. A makeshift roof concealed it from neighboring eyes. When the dice were rolling, kids weren't allowed in the back—no surprise there. But it never stopped me from sneaking in.

Uncle Kenny talked trash whether he was winning or losing. Whenever he got angry, he threatened to "knock niggas into the middle of next week." How strong he must've been to be able to hit someone so hard that they landed on another date.

When one man tried to leave the table with his winnings, Uncle Kenny made another wager: that he could knock him over the table if he didn't continue playing. The game continued.

Uncle Kenny had a "good" job working in sanitation. He drove the truck while the garbage men slung trash bags into the jaws of a massive Tonka truck. Tootsie and his brothers worked with their dad on the weekends. When Uncle Kenny promised to take me with him, I truly felt like a Simmons.

"We have to get up at the crack of dawn," he said.

"Yes, sir."

I planned to show him I was a hard worker in the hope that he would take me with him and his sons regularly. I curled up on their love seat for an early slumber. The lights went out.

"I no wanna go to bed." Tara let the entire household know she detested going to bed early.

"I no wanna go to bed," she whined again.

The Brady Bunch turned into the Waltons, but instead of saying "Goodnight, John-boy," her siblings shouted:

"Shut the hell up, Tara."

"Be quiet, Tara."

"Stop whining, Tara."

"Don't make me come in there with my belt, Tara."

Mom would've administered the leather already. I can't say I would've been opposed to it. Needing relief, I went to the bathroom in their basement, which was next to the kitchen. After the whiz, I went into the kitchen to make a syrup sandwich. All the bread was gone, so a cup of Coca-Cola would have to do. I reached into the cabinet to retrieve an empty cup. Movement caught my eye, and I could see the cup was half-filled with roaches. I dropped the cup, and millions of roaches raced in every direction. I jumped back, then high-stepped out of the kitchen, juiced up without any Coke.

Tara had wound down, and the house fell quiet. When I returned to my quarters, I found Kim passed out in my spot. A tank top barely contained her ta-tas. I shook her to wake her up, but her snoring only magnified. I shook her again. With each jostle, her ta-tas crept closer to exposure. So I vigorously tried to wake her up. But nothing happened. I had to settle for the settee.

When I awoke, the daylight alarmed me since there's no daylight at the crack of dawn. I rose off the settee and searched for Rocky, Kennedy, or Tootsie, but I only found Dee-Dee, Tammy, Tara, and Kim. All the boys were gone, and so was Uncle Kenny. With nowhere to go and nothing to do, I curled up on the empty love seat.

Discarded.

Mrs. Gatlin

Psst, come here," he said.

At the end of the empty hallway in school, in the bathroom's doorway, stood a teenager from the projects. He waved his hand, beckoning me into the bathroom. My hall pass dangled at my side, near my full bladder. He took a step toward me while keeping one foot on the bathroom door as if it might lock behind him. It was my first time seeing him, but I'd heard about what he had done. "I said come here," he said.

I'd known it was a bad idea to stay after school. Now I had to make another decision. And my current predicament stemmed from a bad decision I'd made two days earlier. Here's how that one went:

I stood behind a girl named Tisha, waiting for the "gentle persuasion" (the phrase etched in our teacher's paddle). My fourth-grade teacher, Mrs. Gatlin, resembled a piranha with a ponytail. The youngest of all my teachers, she was quick: quick on her feet, quick to get angry, and quick to strike. She kept us in line with her form of discipline. By the time I'd reached her class, the ruler was ineffective. So Mrs. Gatlin took new measures, putting ten rulers together with rubber bands.

Although I didn't want to see anyone get *rulered* by the little dictator, watching Tisha get popped amused everyone. When Mrs. Gatlin whacked Tisha's hand, Tisha rubbed it on her pant leg and had it ready for another whack instantly. She was so quick on the draw; she must've been a gunslinger in a previous life.

I stuck out my right hand and waited for the shellacking. Mrs. Gatlin eyed a spot on my palm, then shook her head. "Put out your left hand," she said, eliminating any choice I had in the matter. I extended my left, which she grabbed and whacked three times in quick succession, in the same spot, inflicting as much pain as she could. I clenched my teeth as the pain swelled. I held my breath but didn't flinch. She wasn't finished.

Mrs. Gatlin had something in mind that was ten times worse than the ruler. It was the one thing that made me flinch: having to speak in front of the class. I'm sure she knew about my anxiety, and that's why she selected me to participate in a math bee.

Mrs. Gatlin called on a list of potential candidates: Dave Beason, who was brilliant, mainly due to his red hair; Dawn Blakely, who was as smart as she thought she was; Timmy Jenkins, who was slimmer than his chance of winning; Alvin Bussy, a wheezing asthmatic who needed his inhaler after two sit-ups; and Aicha. When Mrs. Gatlin included me in the list, Aicha was my reason for agreeing to do it.

I didn't say much to Aicha because of a blockhead named Brian. They were so close that even his desk touched hers. They both lived in building four, so they strolled home together. Picklehead Brian was getting all the love, but fortunately, his name wasn't on the list for the competition.

The last bell of the day rang, and Dave, Timmy, and Alvin bolted from class. They made it to the corner before being stopped by the crossing guard, which is where I caught them.

"Who y'all running from?' I asked Dave.

"Some kid from the projects beat up Sean."

Dave looked over my shoulder. He always feared something.

"First, it was the Black Spades," I scoffed, referring to the street gang from New York that was supposedly terrorizing school kids.

The crossing guard signaled for us to cross. Dave sprinted down Presidential Boulevard, followed by Timmy and Alvin, leaving me and my doubts in the street.

The following day, Mrs. Gatlin had to confirm our willingness to participate in the math bee. It was my opportunity to ditch it. My athleticism was sufficient for me to be a top pick in sports, but academically I was coming off the bench at best. "Rodney, do you still want to participate?" she asked.

Mrs. Gatlin's tone had changed from the day before; it was filled with doubt. I couldn't blame her since my last academic success had been learning the alphabet. She didn't want me to participate. "Sure," I said.

What did I just say? I nodded to convince myself I could do it. The surprise gave me a burst of energy that inflated my chest. "Does anyone else?" Mrs. Gatlin asked. Brian's hand rose, making my chest sink.

"Raise your hands if you're willing to stay after school and prep for the math bee and earn extra credit," Mrs. Gatlin said. Staying after school was against my religion. There was absolutely no way in hell I was staying. Aicha raised her hand. Then I thought, *I could use some extra credit.*

When the final class bell rang, I stood up, ready to bolt, then realized I had agreed to more torture. Mrs. Gatlin explained how the contest worked and gave us tips. While the other students took notes, I drew "yes" and "no" boxes on my paper. I scribbled potential questions for Aicha, then erased them. With only six students in the classroom, perhaps the building, the only calling I heard came from my bladder. After my third time asking her, Mrs. Gatlin permitted me to use the bathroom.

I pulled the doorknob on the third-floor bathroom, but it was locked, so I headed to the second floor. The wind moaned in the stairwell and sucked the door shut behind me. The bang blasted my eardrums. I skipped down the flight of steps, rattled, and hurried into the hallway.

Soon Mrs. Gatlin would wonder why I was taking so long. What if she let Aicha and the others leave before I returned? Then all of this would have been for nothing. I picked up the pace. And now we're at the point where my story began.

"Pssst, get over here."

The teenage thug Dave had warned me about was staring at me from only fifteen yards away. I stood motionless, facing Boogaloo, a bully from the C.C.P. projects.

"If you don't come in this bathroom, I'm going to get you after school."

What a dumb threat. It was already after school. He meant *after* after school. I backed away from the wild animal without any sudden movements. He looked over his shoulder, making sure there weren't any witnesses. As soon as his eyes left me, I jetted back into the stairwell. Before the door slammed shut, I heard:

"I'm going to get you."

Yeah, but not right now.

Mrs. Gatlin could keep her extra credit. My priority became getting home without "getting got." I sat at the back of the class full of anxiety and urine. *I'm going to get you.* What did he mean? Whatever it meant, I was certain it involved his penis. If he had waited inside the bathroom for another fifteen seconds, until I'd gotten in there, I would've known exactly what he meant.

I watched the door. Dave, Timmy, and Alvin were nose down in math problems. I had to warn them. Clearing my throat got Dave's attention.

"Boogaloo is outside," I mimed.

Dave's puzzled look meant I needed another tactic. I tapped my jaw with my fist, the universal sign for getting "effed up." His jaw dropped, meaning he had gotten the message. And so had Timmy and Alvin. We were united in worry. The bell rang. Time was up.

I tightened my belt, checked my laces, and fastened my pockets. Overtaking Timmy and Alvin would be simple. But Dave was fast, probably due to his Jamaican DNA. I wasn't too worried until I saw that the three of them had already lined up. The last in line was the first to get caught. As the old expression went, "If you slow, you blow."

Conditions had to be favorable for my survival: a green traffic light, no crossing guard, and no Boogaloo. I took my mark, got set, and…I'll be damned. Mrs. Gatlin asked me to dump her pencil shavings into the garbage. *You want me to risk my life over damn pencil shavings?* She was trying to set me up. Before I could dump the shavings, the bell rang. I flew past Mrs. Gatlin's desk with a tailwind that kicked up her papers. Tim's heels and Alvin's elbows dashed in front of me. The traffic light turned yellow. If it turned red, I was done.

Like an impala with a cheetah on his ass, I gunned it. After seconds of running, Alvin reached for his inhaler. I shot past him as quick as the breath of air that he needed. Timmy zipped up the boulevard while Dave held the lead, sailing in the wind. A car pulled into the driveway of building four, stalling them both. They glanced back as I closed in. From their horrid expressions, I knew that Boogaloo was behind me.

Timmy made a hard right toward the entrances to building three. I lived in the building farthest from the school, and on one of the highest floors, miles from safety. Dave hung a right toward building two. Boogaloo didn't go after him; it was clear who he wanted. Gunning toward my lobby, I needed precision in timing to enter the buzz-in security door. A resident needed to be leaving or getting buzzed in at the moment I approached. Otherwise, I'd be trapped in a vestibule with a predator.

I sensed his arm about to grab me, and I dipped my shoulder, then cut a hard right up the sidewalk. An elderly woman waddled toward the door and released it. Dammit! I heaved myself forward up the first landing, then the next, and caught the edge of the metal door with my fingertips, nearly crushing them. I slipped through the door, hoping it would lock behind me. It didn't.

Boogaloo caught the handle before it locked. I couldn't chance the elevator, so I headed toward the stairwell, where people "get got" all the time. After heaving myself up seven flights, I bent over, gasping to fill my lungs with the pissy air. I heard him coming. He hadn't given up; neither could I. With seven flights to go, I grabbed the railing and propelled myself forward. I burst out of the exit on my floor and knocked on our door. I wanted to pound it but was afraid. Howard didn't answer.

What if he's not home? I turned to face Boogaloo, who I was certain would charge out from the exit any second. The door opened and I stumbled backward, greeted by Howard's scowl. A scowl I was thrilled to see. I threw my bookbag aside, ran into the bathroom, and filled the toilet with relief.

My alarm clock the next morning was the pangs in my tummy. The smell of ham and eggs roused me from my sleep. The meat sizzled, and cheese was melted on the heap of eggs sitting on the table as Mom stirred the pot of grits. She made a big breakfast every morning when she worked second shift. At the table, I considered telling her about the bully, but I already knew her solution.

"What's wrong?" Mom asked.

"Uh, nothing."

"I know something happened. Howard said you came home like you were being chased."

How could I tell her I was being bullied on both sides of the door? She buttered the toast, waiting on my response.

"I've been selected to enter into a math bee."

"Wow, a math bee. Is that like a spelling bee?"

I nodded. She spooned scrambled eggs onto a plate next to a slice of ham and buttered grits, then set the plate in front of me.

"When is it?"

"Wednesday. Can you come?"

"I don't know. If I can get off."

She stuffed a thick bologna sandwich wrapped in aluminum foil, plus a box of animal crackers and a no-frills soda, into my lunch bucket.

"If you win, I'll give you ten dollars."

"Ten dollars! Ten whole dollars?"

"Ten whole dollars," Mom said.

Aicha and the other contestants continued staying after school, sharpening their math skills until the day of the contest. Not me. I was first in line to leave, determined to not *get got*. I heard that Boogaloo had caught a boy named Nino in the bathroom. Poor Nino left the bathroom without any visible bruises.

On the day of the math bee, I followed Aicha, Timmy, Alvin, and Dave backstage, where we assembled with the other contestants. We were given seating arrangements and numbers to drape over our shirts—mine was eleven. A teacher went over where to stand and told us to make sure we spoke loudly. The contest began, and that's when number eleven—me—started biting his lips.

There was a panel of three teachers who sat behind microphones at a table offstage. Two of the teachers alternated firing math problems at us, while one held a stopwatch.

"Number eleven, take center stage," a teacher said.

I was certain I knew how to walk. I just had to do it while the whole world watched.

"What's twelve times thirteen?" the teacher asked.

I scanned the front row to see if Mom was in the audience.

"One hundred fifty-six."

"Correct."

I had rubbed the sweat off my palms onto my jeans and returned to my seat before the applause registered. Even Aicha applauded, which stirred hope. As the difficulty of the problems increased, the number of contestants decreased. Dave, Timmy, and Alvin got eliminated. Then only Aicha, Brian, and I were left from our class. Aicha's number was called. "What's twenty-four times eighteen?" she was asked.

I crossed my fingers to help her, but it didn't help. After another round, only Brian, Barry, and I remained. Brian went next and was eliminated. Can't say I was upset about that. "Will the final two contestants step forward for the final round," a teacher said.

From the judge's table, a brilliant trophy was unveiled. Barry had to take the first problem in the elimination round. "What's seventeen times nineteen?" the teacher asked. Barry calculated in his head for a second.

"Three hundred thirteen."

"That's incorrect."

A hush came over the crowd because Barry was favored to win.

"Rodney, if you answer the next equation correctly, you will win the Math bee. What's twenty-three times sixteen?"

"Twenty-three times sixteen," I repeated.

My mind went blank. Seconds chipped away. If I answered wrong, Barry would win because he wouldn't make another mistake. The time keeper's hand crept toward the ceiling. My time had come.

"Three hundred sixty-eight," I finally answered.

"Correct!"

I'd won. Joy overtook my astonishment as I recognized that all the applause was for me. They presented the trophy: a gold angel with large wings. I shielded my eyes from the lights to peer toward the back rows for Mom. Mrs. Gatlin put her hand on my shoulder, saying: "I always knew you could do it."

You ain't no shit. I left her to join my friends backstage. I gave them a look-see at my new lady, then put the trophy in my backpack. When the audience let out, I checked my surroundings before sprinting home. Before I knocked on the door, I pulled the trophy from my bag and reread the placard: *Winner of the Fourth Grade Math Bee.* The door's lock clicked open. I quickly stuffed the lady in my bag. Howard opened the door as if he'd been expecting me.

"What's that?" he asked.

"Oh, nothing."

Discarded.

The Key

During the summer between fifth and sixth grade, we were moving again, and this time without Howard. To make sure he stayed gone this time, mom had gotten insurance in the form of a new man, Freddy. Looks didn't concern Mom. She favored hardworking men; a uniform overrode an asymmetrical face. If they knew how to punch a clock, she would give them the time of day. Freddy wasn't homely, but he hedged his bet by wearing his PSE&G uniform constantly. (PSE&G was our power company.)

Freddy loved laughing. When he cracked a joke, he cackled before anyone else. His infectious laugh forced you to join him. Freddy's favorite expression was three words jumbled into one: "good-gotta-mighty," which I believed meant "good God almighty." If he missed a lottery by one number, it was "good-gotta-mighty"; tasted savory chicken: "good-gotta-mighty"; stubbed a toe: "good-gotta-mighty."

I never corrected Freddy when he called me "Runnie." I figured it was the best he could do with his Southern drawl, plus boys didn't correct men. He walked on the folded-over backs of his shoes, which turned them into slippers. It was obvious he never planned to run.

"Put your stuff in there," Mom said when we got to the new apartment, which was on North First Street in Paterson. "That's your room."

"My room?"

My room was off the kitchen next to the living room, snug, with a small window. It had an intimate view of the cracked siding on the neighboring house, which was only a long arm's length away. I dropped my boxes on the linoleum floor, dug into one of them, and pulled out my prized possession. I placed it on the dresser, then took a step back to make sure it was centered. The little gold angel stood alone on the bureau. Now it was home.

Tasha's room was next to mine, while Mom and Freddy's was in the back. The bathroom, located in the hallway *outside* the apartment, required getting used to. Someone could easily break in downstairs and hide in the hallway. I worried that while I was copping a squat, an attacker would kick in the bathroom door and think: *I really scared this guy.*

My room wasn't actually mine. Tasha splayed her dolls on my floor and shoved my Stretch Armstrong underneath the bed. I guess he didn't get along with Barbie. If I sat on the bed, she sat on the bed as if we were connected at the hip. My sister would do anything for me except stay out of my freakin' room.

A visit to the dentist's office one time revealed the strength of our connection. My tooth needed removing, initially a DIY project for Mom. First, she had tried to yank it with rusty pliers. When that failed, she had tied one end of a string around my tooth and the other around a doorknob.

"Ready?" she said.

"Uh, not really."

She slammed the door. The string broke, along with my confidence in her decision making. After another round of what could easily be considered blunt-force trauma, she decided to take me to the dentist. The dentist observed the crumbled remains of my cuspid.

"Wow, this tooth has really been beaten up," he said.

"How much for a tetanus shot?' Mom asked.

The dentist's assistant rolled over his metal tray. He uncovered the long needles, hacking knives, and miniature saws, and I thought: *Finally, someone reasonable.* The dentist swabbed a bitter substance on my gums, telling me: "This is anesthesia; it will take the pain away." I pointed to my sister. "Her?"

No one laughed, but I thought it was funny. Pushing my head back, the dentist gripped my tooth with pliers and yanked. The high-pitched scream that followed startled the dentist, Mom, and me. Tasha cupped her mouth to muffle her scream. The pain apparently had jumped from my jaw to my sister's. The dentist giggled as if he'd sniffed the laughing gas. His assistant gave Tasha a sucker and a few encouraging words to console her about the pain *she* was going through while I sat in the chair, losing blood and patience.

The dead-end block of North First Street bustled. Mismatched multifamily houses lined the street, with cracked windows that leaked rhythm and blues. Brown girls played double Dutch, and Black boys flipped on torn mattresses. The block partied as I watched the summer fun from the backseat. Freddy's beige Bonneville would break through touch football games like the icebreaker I needed.

I considered introducing myself to one of my neighbors, but I was certain he planned to shank me. His uncombed hair and snotty nose gave him a crazed look. He would stare at me without blinking from his stoop. He was part of a huge family, who all wore at least one Band-Aid each. For reasons I could only speculate on, they never left the porch. I guessed they were already practicing house arrest.

The stench of stagnation crinkled my nose. One day I discovered an access to the Passaic River at the end of the block. The ground mushed and gushed under my sneakers. I leapfrogged over the muddy embankment, landing on boards, dry patches, and doll heads. A baby carriage drifted by. What if there was a baby inside? A little Black Moses. The thought made me laugh.

A huge water rat swam toward a pack of cigarettes. Must've had a stressful day. Another rat sighting facilitated my decision to leap-frog my ass back home. The river was full of rats, and so was North First Street. The only difference was that the ones in the streets were two-legged.

Skull and Celeste lived in a two-family house that faced ours. Skull lived on the first floor, Celeste on the second. Skull's pop-lock-ing skills made him popular, while Celeste's notoriety came natu-rally. Her boobs could be seen from across the street, I was certain.

Next door to Skull and Celeste lived two caramel-colored sisters who were rarely seen but constantly sought after, especially by the Johnson brothers. The six Johnson boys lived at the top of the block in more ways than one.

When Freddy's fifteen-year-old son, Binky, walked through the door with a suitcase one day, I realized how little I knew about Freddy. Was Binky moving in? After our introduction, Mom offered him something to eat while I stood guard by my room.

"Put your bags in Rodney's room," Mom said.

Really? Binky dropped his gym bag near my bed and gave my Sesame Street comforter the side-eye. I'd been meaning to get a new one. *Don't get too comfortable, slick,* I thought. *This ain't Mr. Rogers' neighborhood; this is Mr. Rodney's neighborhood.*

At dinner that night, I watched Binky while he chewed on the last bite of the last piece of chicken. I looked for a resemblance between him and Freddy. The freckled face and bowl cut made

Binky unique, in my opinion. He pushed away from the table, stuck a lollipop in his mouth, and grabbed a football from his bag. He stopped at the door. "You coming?"

Hell, yeah.

Old Cadillacs, Chevrolets, and other heaps lined both sides of the street, making for a narrow football field. The dead-end street kept traffic to a minimum. Binky rounded up eight guys for a four-on-four game of touch football, which included Skull. Binky played steady quarterback. His marksmanship made his passes easy to catch. As his confidence in my ability increased, so did the heat on his passes. I ran across the middle, and he darted a pass that stuck in the chest. It stung like hell, but I held on to it. "I'm going to call you 'John Jefferson,'" Binky said.

Celeste and the caramel sisters joined the sidelines. The Johnson brothers waited to play next. We huddled up and Binky drew up a play that would earn me respect. Binky took out his lollipop, using the handle to draw up the play on his palm. "You go short. You cut across the middle," Binky said to Skull. He looked at me and waved the lollipop. "And you go for the bomb."

The end of a Plymouth was the line of scrimmage. I peeked over to see if Celeste was still watching. She was. "Hike," Binky called out.

I sprinted deep. Binky pump-faked before launching a rocket with a rainbow trajectory. I had to speed up to catch it. Looking over my shoulder as the football spiraled, I stretched out my arms as the leather floated into my fingertips. Victory was mine once again. Until everything went black.

When I came to, I saw that Binky, Skull, the Johnson brothers, the Caramel sisters, and Celeste were standing over me.

"You OK?" Binky said.

"What happened?"

"You ran into a van."

I stood up for a second and wobbled. Binky shouldered me to our porch, where Mom awaited. "Cars are supposed to hit you; you're not supposed to hit them," Mom said in jest.

Binky bust a gut laughing. I heard others laugh. *I'm glad to know my injury caused so much joy.* Even Tasha laughed while rubbing her forehead.

Although Binky eventually left our apartment, his presence lasted like the dent my face left in that van. There was one benefit to running into a parked vehicle. I earned a nickname. I became "the kid who slammed face-first into parked vans." I admit it was a little long.

One day not long after Binky left, Celeste waved for me to come over to her patio. It was a pass that hit me in the chest. I zipped across the street without looking; if a car had been coming, my popularity would've soared. I stopped at the gate, double-checking with her for permission to enter. She assured me with another wave. She sat cross-legged on her perch. White jean shorts revealed her slim legs, glistening from Vaseline. Her peachy tank top held so much promise, giving me a ray of hope. I tried playing it cool by leaning against the wall, but a nail pierced my back. I slid over to the banister, giving Celeste a wide smile to cover the pain.

I wanted to know if everything I had imagined about Celeste was true. She talked. I listened. Time eased by. It had to be nearing dinnertime; soon, Mom or Tasha would come looking. When I stood up to go, Celeste followed me onto the sidewalk. She grabbed my hand and kindled something in me with her gaze. Her hazel eyes gave me something I had only experienced once before: a flash of significance. And we kissed.

Clothes make the man, baby! I'd heard that phrase numerous times. My wardrobe became a matter of life and death. I was getting ready to start at a new school that fall but couldn't attend a new school without new gear. I begged Mom to buy me clothes with recognizable names, and to my astonishment, she did. I laid my school clothes across the bed, smacking my hands together and giving a big nod of approval. The only stain in the lineup was my no-name sneakers.

I went over to the Passaic River and tried to skip rocks into it, but the dark water buried them immediately. I couldn't focus on skipping anyway; my thoughts were on Celeste. Other than the foul fishy odor and an occasional rat, the river access was a good spot to chill or kiss or commit a murder. I had just heaved a rock as far as I could when Kevin Johnson crept up behind me.

"Hey, you that kid that tried to move a van with his face?" Kevin asked.

"Yes."

"And you didn't lose any teef?"

I shook my head. He seemed disappointed after revealing a four-tooth smile.

"You want to see something cool?" Kevin asked.

"Sure."

As long as there's no bathroom involved, I thought. I followed him up the street into his backyard, where guys were shooting dice. "Those are my brothers, cockeyed Alvin, Melvin, and Trouble," he said.

I respect a guy whose name is also a warning. The only one who looked at me was Alvin, I assumed. Kevin pointed to the reason he'd brought me to his backyard. Built in a stumpy tree with random pieces of plywood and two-by-fours was a treehouse.

It hovered an astonishing two feet above the ground. I entered after climbing the one step. Inside it creaked and rocked with each step. I was certain we were going fall all twenty-four inches to our death. "I painted it myself," Kevin said.

Did you use a mop? I thought. Kevin babbled nonstop about his brothers as I contemplated an exit strategy.

"My brother Melvin brings his girls to the treehouse all the time."

"Really?" *Tell me more.*

After my treehouse visit, I stood in front of our apartment strip searching myself for my keys. I was a loser. If Mom sent me to the store with ten dollars and a list of items, I'd return without the items, without the list, and without the ten-dollar bill. If it could be lost, I'd lose it. It infuriated Mom. I was the reason Child Protective Services was created. I lost my keys so often, she invented ways to prevent me from losing them. First, she tried hanging them around my neck. When that didn't work, she safety-pinned them to my shirt. When that didn't work, she threatened to shove them up my ass. Luckily, she didn't.

If I couldn't find them, an ass whooping would find me. So on this day, I waited outside, hoping I could catch Freddy leaving. I rang the bell. Freddy opened the door and paused as if he was waiting for an explanation.

"Whatcha thinking about?" he asked.

"Nothing."

"You must be thinking about something. Know how I know?"

"How?"

"I smell a peanut roasting."

Freddy laughed at his own joke, and I encouraged him. Relieved, I went into my room, plopped down on my bed, and contemplated the next kiss while my golden angel watched over me.

The copper sunset at Garret Mountain Reservation marked a new semester at school and the end of summer vacation. From the overlook, you could see the New York City skyline and much of Route 80. Couples gazed through the metered binoculars, maybe looking into their future. Garret Mountain overlooked the Towers, where we lived. I could see my past on the balcony of 14C. I missed Dave, Alvin, Timmy, and Aicha. I wondered about Mietta and if she had checked somebody else's box. I thought about public school number twelve, where I was headed, and if I would get along with the students there.

Mom rolled up the picnic blanket, and I carried her boom box. Freddy had driven us to the park for our final outing before school started. When we got back home and Freddy parked the car, I hopped out, ready to relax in my room. Then I remembered the key situation and fell back. Freddy inserted his key into the dead bolt.

"Good-gotta-mighty! Wait here."

Our apartment had been broken into.

Freddy searched each room before the rest of us entered, then we fanned out, looking for missing items. The thieves had taken the toaster and the TV. Nothing had been stolen from Tasha's room. I flipped the light in my room and discovered the worst. I yanked open my drawers to find that all my new clothes had been stolen. They'd left behind my no-name sneakers.

I sank deep into my bed and closed my eyes. Mom's and Freddy's frenetic voices receded. Then I sat up and turned toward the dresser. Damn. My angel was gone.

Resolved to catch the thieves, I headed to the front porch for a stakeout. How would Encyclopedia Brown solve the mystery of the stolen Lee jeans and math bee trophy? I searched for answers and for Celeste, whom I hadn't seen since our kiss.

I thought about how many crimes go unsolved and how trying to solve the case was hopeless until cockeyed Alvin strutted down the street wearing my Lees. They were high-waters on him, stopping four inches above his ankles. I rushed upstairs to tell Mom, who was now alone in the house watching *Guiding Light*. She trailed me to the living room window. A male figure had entered our gate, then disappeared under the porch roof before we could see his face. The steps creaked as he approached our door. We scrambled into the kitchen, where we waited, watching the door. He didn't knock; he only listened. Mom crept over to the kitchen drawer and grabbed a Ginsu meat cleaver. A key was inserted into the lock. The dead bolt wasn't engaged. Nothing would stop his entry. The doorknob began turning. Mom raised her cleaver. I tiptoed to the door before he could open it and bolted the top lock. The door jerked while Mom and I shuddered. A final yank signaled his defeat. The steps creaked again, and we hustled to the front window to see Melvin Johnson crossing the street to meet up with his brother Alvin.

Mom sparked a cigarette, took long drags, and tapped the ashes into an ashtray next to the knife. I began to relax without the aid of nicotine until Mom asked:

"Where are your keys?"

I had camped out on the porch hoping to catch another winning pass from Celeste. The game ended when Mom sounded the dinner alarm. Celeste walked out of her house and glided down her steps. I waved, then hopped down to the sidewalk. I had just opened the latch on our gate when she finally looked at me. I waved again, but she turned her head and kept walking as if she didn't see me. With no idea what to do, I settled on looking stupid.

We were moving again. The U-Haul truck was packed and ready to go.

Mom, Tasha, and I waited quietly in Mom's car while Freddy padlocked the truck. Tasha's normal animation was suppressed by an impending ass whooping. Freddy had moved the stove and found a surprise behind it: the rotting vegetables Tasha had been dumping there. That's why she always had a clean plate.

The U-Haul truck blocked my view of Celeste's house. I waited for Freddy to move the truck, wondering if Celeste would at least wave goodbye. Mom pulled ahead, leading the U-Haul truck up North First Street. There was no last-minute surprise.

There are no cul-de-sacs in the hood, only dead ends. We'd traded one dead end for another that was only seven blocks away. We'd spend the next seven years in that one. Mom must've learned you can't always run away from trouble.

Discarded.

The Fellas

A crowd gathered in my peripheral vision at the corner of North Fourth Street and Barnert Place, excited for the pending fight. "Get him, Mark. Get him," the kids from school twelve shouted—"him" being me. *How did I end up here?* The thought flashed through my mind. It didn't matter now. The only thing that did matter was protecting my chin from the haymakers about to be thrown by Mark Foreman.

The brawny kid bobbed his head like a Tuesday-night fighter, making me wish I had a Saturday Night special (a popular handgun). Instincts were all I had. They had to be enough. Every time Mark landed a punch, school twelve cheered, egging him on. I held my fists in front of my face, waiting for another jab. He lunged with a hook. I ducked, then countered with a straight right to his jaw. I stunned him and shocked myself.

"Oooooh." School twelve disapproved of my score. Mark felt his jaw, then switched gears. Shit just got real. My long, broomstick arms kept him cautious. I threw a confident hook that missed. He counterattacked by grabbing my legs. *Wait, is this legal?* He scooped me up in the air...

Before I continue, let me explain something. In our hood, there were a few ways to determine the victor of a fight. If you got knocked out, the fight was over. If you got pummeled into submission, the fight was over. And if you got slammed, the freakin' fight was over.

…and slammed me on the concrete. The back-breaking concrete.

"Oooooooh, he got slammed," the school twelvers taunted.

They cheered their boy. I dusted off, congratulated Mark (in my mind), and stepped off. *At least I got one good lick in*, I said to console myself, an attempt that fell as flat as I had fallen.

We had moved into apartment D of a lone two-story, fourteen-unit brick rowhouse apartment building at the end of a dead-end street. Every four apartments shared a narrow front porch supported by iron railings. I had to share a room with Tasha, who was somewhere wondering why her back was hurting—given how she seemed to feel what I did. I climbed into the top bunk and replayed the crowd cheering for Mark over and over in my head until I conked out.

Laura King, a Nabisco coworker of my Mom's, had recommended the apartment. She lived in the building with her two sons, Eric and Squanky. Laura introduced me to them, so my smashing-face-first-into-parked-vans technique for making friends was unnecessary.

"Introduce him to your friends," Laura told her boys.

Eric introduced me to Alfie, who lived in the apartment above them; A. T., the son of a preacher man; and Kenny Pickett, a kid whose glasses were *Guinness Book of World Records* thick. I liked him immediately.

"You play football?" Alfie said.

"Not in the street," I said.

"He better be able to catch with those long-ass arms," Eric said.

"They don't call me 'John Jefferson' for nothing," I said.

We warmed up on the patio. Eric tossed me the football. I flung it to A. T., who chucked it to Kenny. The patio's short size prevented bomb passes. I didn't mind at all.

When the streetlights came on, Freddy called out: "Runnie! Time to eat, Runnie."

"Runnie?" Eric said.

I zipped the football back to Eric before heading home.

"See you tomorrow, Runnie," Eric said.

The neighborhood was quiet in "the Dead End"—the nickname given to my new hood. Eric and Alfie stood on their porch while Kenny, A. T., and I sat on the stoop below them, arrested by the ruckus.

"Hold the goddamn door, Turner," a woman screamed.

"Carol, calm down now," Turner said.

"Don't you tell me to fuckin' calm down, Turner."

Carol, a frail-looking woman who couldn't curl a toothpick, was draped in pearls. Turner sucked on a cigarette while fumbling with a lamp cord that dangled down to his pigeon toes.

"Keith, Jaima, get y'all asses up here and help Turner," Carol said.

"Looks like you got some rowdy ones movin' in, Rod," A. T. said.

"I'm glad they moving in next to y'all, with that mouth," Eric said.

"It can't be worse than yours," I replied.

Kenny snickered.

Keith "brought his narrow ass" following his mamma's order. He fought to carry a wooden box and noticed us watching. He stopped and stared back. Easing up behind him was Jaima—whose ass was not narrow.

Alfie and Eric, the Romeos of our clique, stood up to get a better view. A. T., Kenny, and I remained seated. The urge to use the bathroom overcame me, so I quit the group and pimp-strolled toward home.

Was it an attempt to boost my chances with Jaima? Not really. I was just goofing around, but it backfired when she appeared at the top of the landing. The fellas were watching. At least when Celeste had dissed me, there had been no witnesses. Jaima smiled. I knew the smile wasn't for me—it couldn't be—but I stole it anyway and tucked it in my pocket. I slowed my pace, giving her time to enter her apartment, ensuring I wouldn't have to say anything to her. Yet.

A few days later, Keith had draped a pair of Black Dragon nun-chucks around his neck. His baggy karate gi made him appear stout. From the opposite end of the apartment building, he kicked air and howled the same way Bruce Lee did when he killed Bolo. Keith was sending us a warning.

Kenny bounced a ball off the side of the building, playing catch with himself, while A. T. and I sat on the stoop. Eric tossed a trash bag into the garbage shed, then put the latch back in place.

"What is he doing?" Kenny said.

"Those nunchucks weigh more than he does," I said.

"You think he know karate?" A. T. asked.

"Hell, no. He probably got those nunchucks from the Chinese restaurant," Eric said.

Keith punched the air and howled again like he'd stepped on a nail. He probably didn't know kung fu, but I'd watched too many karate movies to risk it. Who wears a karate uniform and doesn't know karate?

Our shared porch made it easy to run into Jaima, especially when I waited for her. We often "coincidentally" left for school at the same time, even when she was late. Being late didn't stop her from stopping at the corner store, where she stocked up on her Chick-O-Sticks, Bazooka gum, and Pop Rocks candy. She would dump the packet of Pop Rocks on her tongue, which made her smile sizzle until we reached the playground.

School twelve's square playground would fill in a half hour before the lineup bell. Eighth graders ruled the yard, while the first graders ran free. Before Jaima, I would arrive early to play Garmen, which was a better version of tag. Jaima, like most girls, didn't play Garmen. The girls preferred double Dutch and stepping.

Stepping wasn't a game but a dance or cheer or—if you were a dad, a display of your daughter's loose morals. The girls would gather in a circle, with each girl waiting her turn to get nasty, singing, "I'm going to shake my booty, pop my cootie, and git on down, git on down, an git back up." They cheered each other on. Some girls were prohibited from stepping by their parents. I wonder why. Occasionally a father would surprise his daughter, catch her *popping her cootie*, and commence *popping that ass*. Although Jaima had come from Governor Street, a street known for tricks and chalk outlines, she never stepped. That booty didn't shake for anyone, to my chagrin.

My friendship with Jaima led to one with Keith. He and I got tighter than their welfare budget. Little John, the neighborhood pushover, once confronted Keith and wrestled him to the ground.

Who wears a karate uniform and doesn't know karate? Turns out, Keith. After that, Keith became an easy mark.

Cracking, busting, or hiking was a sport: a dangerous sport that killed self-esteem. Our brand of busts started with "you big..." "You big cockeyed eyes like a pair of dice." "You big bubble-headed snaggletooth."

Everyone and their mother were targets. "I saw your mother running barefoot from the police, carrying a floor-model TV, singing 'We Shall Overcome Someday.'"

Jokes targeted insecurities or created them. Even the thickest skin would crack under fire, releasing tears or fists.

A kid named Junnie had a right calf that was smaller than his left due to a childhood cast. Another kid, Chris McKinney, once bust on Junnie so hard, he went in the house. We were certain he was going to cry. Because he'd made it to the house didn't mean he was safe.

"Junnie, if you're going to hang yourself, stand on your good leg. And don't forget to leave a note," Chris said.

"Junnie's note would read: 'I'd still be here if I had a better comeback,'" I said.

Some situations warranted more than a good comeback—they warranted revenge.

One cloudy afternoon, Jaima and I had just reached the landing of the steps when Keith rushed toward us, a vein bulging on his temple.

"What happened?" Jaima asked.

"They effing play too much."

He ripped open the door and ran into their apartment. "Don't do nothing stupid, Keith," Jaima said. She hurried after him. I hesitated, uncertain if I should follow Jaima. Keith came out and rumbled back down the stairs and kicked the apartment door open, gripping one end of his nunchucks. The other end banged against the rail as he raced by us. Before he hopped off the porch, Jaima caught the loose end of the nunchucks, then snatched them from her brother's clutch. Keith leaped at his sister, grabbing for his weapon. Jaima strong-armed him. "Calm down, Keith," she said.

A group of fellas ascended from Kenny's basement nearby, laughing as they spilled onto the sidewalk. "What happened?" I asked Keith. He wouldn't say, and his frustration bubbled into tears. He darted back into his apartment. The guys—Eric, A. T., Kenny, Squanky, and Cool C.—were still giggling as I approached.

"What happened?" I asked them.

Kenny shook his head. "Somehow, a game of pool ended with Keith being held down." He burst into laughter again. "And they held him down right. And Chris had this banana, and..."

"What?" I said.

"There was no penetration," Chris declared.

As if that was any better. Then again, I guess it was. But still. Who does that?

Jaima was waiting for me on our porch, and I walked back over there.

"What they say?" she asked.

"Um, looks like a prank that went south," I said. *Or up north, depending on how you look at it.*

"I'm calling Raina," Jaima said.

Raina, her older sister, still lived on the notorious Governor Street. If she were to come… I looked toward the fellas, who were choosing sides for a football game.

"I'm sure they was just horsing around," I said.

Jaima tilted her head and dismissed me with a sharp suck of her teeth. She leaned over the banister, looking toward the fellas.

"Y'all going to get yours!" Jaima warned.

Keith rumbled down the steps.

"Raina's on her way," he said. That big peanut-head joker had called her already. I had been wondering who Raina resembled— if she was an older version of Jaima or a younger version of her mother, Ms. Carol. I was about to find out.

I joined the others for the game. Chris left, but the other fellas and I remained in the courtyard. We had just finished the football game when Raina arrived.

"Which one of you punk bitches put their fucking hands on my little brother?" She was the spitting image of Ms. Carol.

Keith and Jaima followed Raina as she marched toward us. The fellas gathered near Eric's porch while I stood near the wall between them and my porch. Raina held one hand behind her back as she approached.

"Y'all ain't got nuttin' to say now, huh?"

Her eyes shifted from Eric to Kenny to A. T. to me, searching for a response or a target.

"One missing," Keith said.

"Y'all bitch-asses not so tough now," Raina said.

No one said anything.

"Raina, get yo ass back here now," Ms. Carol said from the porch. She marched off our porch, tying her robe.

Raina brandished her weapon, a butcher's knife as long as her arm.

"Put your hands on my brother again, see what happens," she threatened.

Raina and her family receded in silence. Ms. Carol pointed upstairs as her children walked by. After she shut their door, the chatter commenced.

"Man, I would've whooped her ass if she'd came closer," Eric said.

We all laughed.

Discarded.

The Holy Ghost

Iput God in a dilemma every Saturday night by praying that I wouldn't have to go to church on Sunday. My prayers went unanswered, and I was sent to Serenity Baptist Church. Every freakin' Sunday.

Religion puzzled me. Was I supposed to love God or fear him? Could I do both? The Son, the Father, and the Holy Ghost? Out of the three, the Holy Ghost received the least amount of attention from our preacher. Maybe that's why she showed up in church and made people shout—to get more respect. The good preacher shouted for glory while the congregation testified. What did that feel like? I believed in God for one reason. It was safe. Why gamble with your soul? That's a game you don't want to lose, else you will burn for a really, really long time.

Keith and I would stop at Roger's corner store before church, the highlight of our Sunday morning. The silver coins meant for offerings bought Now & Laters and Jolly Ranchers. Keith had a penchant for licorice, or as he called it, "lik-a-wish."

Serenity Baptist Church stood out in the residential area due to its money-green color. Three sections of pews formed a semicircular pattern from the podium, and vibrations stemmed from the pulpit. One Sunday, Keith followed me into an empty pew nearest the exit. Since it wasn't a holiday, the church wasn't crowded. The first signs of a long sermon and we would be ghosts. More members filed in, mostly older women wearing clothes made from carpet and stockings thicker than casts.

I envied the certitude of the huge-hatted women, who rocked in their seats while staving off the heat with their Dr. Martin Luther King fans. They showed up faithfully, like the gout in their toes on days promising rain. They hummed along to the music before one note was played. They sat close to the pulpit, and closer to Jesus, in God's V.I.P. section.

The sermon started with opening remarks from one of the big hats. I hoped she would lead us into song, and she did. The choir was the entertainment that highlighted the service and made my spirit do a two-step. The choir opened up with "Soon and Very Soon," and the entire congregation sang along.

I flipped through the hymn book, searching for the lyrics while the straw donation basket made its rounds. I arrived at the lyrics too late, and the offering basket arrived too early. I delivered my change underhandedly. "First a few announcements," a deacon said.

"Who put pennies in the basket?" I feared he'd say.

A butterball of a woman, in an orange dress and matching bright hat, squeezed into our pew, blocking our exit. *For God's sake.* The congregation applauded as the pastor took the pulpit. Ms. Orange Dress, the woman who had us pinned in, thumbed through her Bible and grabbed a fan.

"Preach," she praised.

A long sermon was in the making. At the back of the center pew, a young lady was tinkering with a Rubik's Cube. She'd had the audacity to bring a Rubik's Cube to the house of the Lord. I was annoyed. Why hadn't I thought of that?

If we were going to sneak out, it had to be before the organist started. Once he started striking those chords, emphasizing the sermon, the Holy Ghost would start uplifting and uprooting the big hats from their seats. Mom often quizzed me about the lesson, so I hung out long enough to hear the beginning. The preacher spoke about Samson, a strong dude with long hair who was set up by a chick who scalped him. In return, he pulled down giant pillars and killed everybody and himself. Moral of the story: Women will cut you if you turn your back on them. Got it.

The organist strummed a note that reverberated from the pulpit straight into the souls of the congregation. Damn. It was too late. The Holy Ghosts were alerted. You always knew who would catch the ghost. They were the ones who "amen"-ed every syllable the preacher made. At least that's what I thought until the girl with the Rubik's Cube started spasming. I thought: *Damn, she is really happy to solve that puzzle.*

"Keith, see that girl right there?" I said.

"The one jumping around?" Keith said.

"Yeah, she was just playing with a Rubik's Cube."

Keith didn't give a damn. Something else had captured his attention. Ms. Orange Dress had leaped out of her seat.

"Jeeeeeeezzus," she said.

With raised arms and a bobbing head, she surrendered to God. The sermon revved into another gear as the pastor whipped the church into a frenzy.

"Hallelujah!" the congregation shouted.

Ms. Orange Dress stood up. She started heaving as if the Holy Ghost was using the Heimlich maneuver on her. She was off-balance, coming toward us in the pew, completely out of control.

She'd gone full-blown Holy Ghost and was headed straight toward Keith. Four hundred pounds of "hallelujah" were about to come crashing down on Keith, and he knew it. He needed to know more than karate to deal with the threat. He needed to know sumo wrestling. He swallowed hard, knowing his sixty-pound frame would be crushed under her weight. Keith's anxiety turned to fear, then panic.

"Jeeeeeezzus, oh Jeeeeeeezus."

"Oh God, no," Keith said.

"Jeeeeeezus, oh Jeeeeeeezus."

Within two feet—striking distance—she forced Keith into action. Keith gave me one final look, then grabbed the back of the pew with both hands.

"Jeeeeeeezus, oh Jeeeeeeezus."

She was within inches now. Keith threw one foot on the back of the pew, readying himself, then hopped over the pew, landing into the next row.

"Jeeeeeezus, oh Jeeezus."

The woman toppled, landing on me. I used my forearm to create shelter; it seeped deep into her rib cage as she otherwise smothered me. Ushers scooted down the aisle to disentangle us. Ms. Orange Dress regained her composure readily, but it took me a minute to regain mine. Twenty minutes later, I was still laughing at Keith. Evil glances came from Ms. Orange Dress and the big-hatted people. Even the girl with the Rubik's Cube stared at me, but I couldn't stop laughing.

I tapped Keith on the back of his leg and stood up before the end of the sermon. I waited for Ms. Orange Dress to move her legs aside, then exited the church regardless of who was watching.

Discarded.

Paper

Anthony Robinson was cooler than the Marlboro Man. I'll never forget the day he joined our six-grade classroom. The way his gray-on-blue Pumas matched his outfit was on the money. Their fat red laces matched the line running down his Puma sweatsuit. Extra dope. After checking out his dope sneakers, I hid my no-name sneakers (japs) under my seat. Mom bought my sneakers out of a bin at the Pathmark supermarket—an impulse purchase, like her Juicy Fruit and *TV Guide*.

Anthony's chest beefed up his tank top and bulged out toward his hairy armpits. He would have been in the class with the ruffians if he hadn't been left back. That's how he'd ended up in our class—well, Mrs. Nelson's class. He didn't belong with the roughnecks; he belonged with us. Anthony was respected by the block and had a rep with the ladies. Being his classmate had its advantages.

One day after school, I crossed North Fifth Street, heading to Roger's to buy flour and Raid. The combination made it seem as if we wanted to bake roaches. Of the many porches between North Fifth and North Fourth, one towered above the rest. From their perch, the two hotties, Morny and Raquel, looked down at everyone on their way to Roger's. It took twenty-five steps to reach their porch, two of my lucky numbers.

Many fifty-cent Romeos desiring to knock Raquel and Morny off their roost would float up that staircase to face the smart-mouthed duo. And just as many would stumble back down after falling flat on their face.

I laid the spray can facedown on the counter at Roger's. The world didn't need to know our issues. I could hear the cracks: "You big roach-infested-house-having…" Barbara, the clerk, missed the hint completely.

"How many roaches do y'all have?" she asked. "You might want to try a defogger. You know what those are?"

I nodded even though I didn't.

"Tell your momma we have d-CON; it works just as good."

Thanks for the pesticide lesson. Now may I have a bullet to the head to go with it, please?

"Can I have a brown bag?" I said.

Anthony was chilling on the corner when I exited the store, finishing off a Mellow Yello. I gave him a pound as he walked by. He nuzzled up to the store's facade behind me, pulled from his pants what I assumed was a baby seal, then started peeing.

Oh, we just peeing out in the open? I thought.

Looking over his shoulder, he asked: "What you up to today?"

Erasing this imagery from my memory.

"I see Morny and Raquel's hanging out," I said.

"Oh yeah. You going up?"

"Um, I don't know."

I knew damn well I wasn't going up. The stream of urine headed toward my sneakers. I stepped aside so it could flow into the sewer. Anthony shook off the excess, then zipped up. "Let's go," he said.

I followed Anthony up Morny and Raquel's steps, cozied myself in the corner of their porch, and looked down at the sidewalk.

It would have been cool if one of the fellas had been walking by. Anthony settled between the two girls, who were eyeing me over and not in a good way. They were about to start busting. I forced a giggle for Morny's over-the-top jokes. Raquel had a scar, a burn mark, on her face that gave her the look of someone who would cut you as fast as kiss you. It made her wildly alluring. Her wisecracks were quiet but deadly, like high blood pressure.

"Your sneakers are fresh to death," Morny told Anthony.

"What kind of sneakers are those, Rodney?" Morny said.

My blood pressure jumped thirty points.

"FootJoys," I mumbled.

"More like eye pains," Raquel said.

Anthony cracked up. I chuckled, but my laugh was cheaper than my shoes. I perused my mind for a decent comeback, but they were all too mean. "Did you mistake lye for lotion?" would've eliminated any chance of getting with her.

I figured the busts wouldn't last long. I figured wrong. My FootJoys inspired dozens of cracks—even Anthony joined in. After I endured all of their cheap sneaker jokes, I felt a sense of relief because there was nothing left to crack on. Then Morny asked, "What's in the bag?"

My cue to leave. Another Romeo crushed.

It was time for me to earn dough, make moolah, get some ducats, so I could ditch the FootJoys and buy some decent sneakers. The money Freddy gave me for taking out the trash wasn't enough. My best option for getting paper was getting a paper route.

A few days later, Mr. Blake, the paper man, sat on the edge of our sofa, leaning over the newspapers and plastic bags displayed on the coffee table. Mom stood over us as Mr. Blake demonstrated how to roll the papers and stuff them in the bags.

"These bags are for when it rains," he said.

The papers smelled fresh as if they had just been printed.

"Now, let me see you do it," Mr. Blake said.

I should've studied for this. I guess he considered it on-the-job training. I did as the man said. He oozed with enthusiasm: "Yeah, that's it." He pulled from his leather satchel a list of addresses. "The papers have to be delivered every morning before school."

Before school? Well, that would mean waking up at...?

"Is that a problem?" Mr. Blake asked.

"No," I said.

He stood, shook Mom's hand, and patted me on the back.

"Follow me to my car," he told me. "I forgot something."

I followed him to his car.

"For every dollar and twenty cents you collect, you keep forty cents."

"What if they don't pay?" I said.

He stopped in front of a van. I thought he'd said "car." He stuck his key in the back door, then yanked it open, revealing...*all the kids he had kidnapped and tortured.* My fears were getting the best of me.

But no, there were just bundles of papers lining the back, along with empty pizza boxes and soda cans. Carpet quieted his footsteps as he climbed in. If he asked me to follow him, I would slam the door on him and jet. He pulled something out of a bag, saying: "Here, you'll need this."

He chucked me a cloth sack that read "*Herald News.*"

"People pay. This business is built on trust. Can I trust you?" he said.

"Yeah."

"We'll see."

The headlines flashed by over the weeks: Franklin Jacobs, a hometown hero, was considering a return to the Olympics. Jimmy Carter was losing his battle of fighting inflation. Ronald Reagan was threatening world peace. The rookie Magic Johnson had made the all-star basketball team. I only glimpsed each headline before rolling up each paper with a rubber band and bouncing out the door. My route was seven long blocks and all hill.

One day early on, Keith sat on his stoop eating as I hit the landing with an empty sack.

"You ever try collecting money from people who lived in the ghetto?" I asked him.

Keith shoved another piece of toast with jelly in his mouth and shook his head. I mimicked Richard Pryor: "It's harder than Chinese arithmetic."

Keith didn't get it. He hated math as much as I hated asking adults for payment. Even men with good jobs, like Mr. Moore, delayed payment.

"Come back next week. I'll pay you for both weeks," Mr. Moore had said.

It's only a dollar twenty, you big nine-foot-two broke-ass, no-change-having… Some clients gave half—half of a dollar twenty. *This ain't a damn layaway plan. Now I have to keep a record of your half-assed payment?*

Mr. Blake counted the money I collected on our coffee table, cupped his hand, and pulled his portion into his collection box, a ritual he would perform every weekend. I scooped up the few worn dollars, quarters, and nickels left over. I stashed my money in a tube sock underneath my mattress. I calculated it would take three weeks for me to save the forty-two dollars I needed.

After a prosperous Saturday, my pockets bulged and jingled from the quarters I had collected. I whipped the empty sack around my back, creating a breeze to stave off the day's mugginess. Many of my clients had paid, and even the previously delinquent clients were caught up on their balances.

An orange soda and a bag of chips from Roger's had my name on them. I put two quarters on the counter, turned to leave, and heard an unexpected explosion. Then an android warned, "Intruder alert. Intruder alert."

Roger had installed a new video arcade game, Berzerk. A six-inch joystick jutted out from the machine. I squeezed the bottom of the bag of chips to pop it open and commence to crunching. A stick man ran through a maze while firing laser bullets at robots. He had to escape the maze before a giant bouncing smiley face killed him. I dug in my pocket and slid one of my many quarters into the machine.

The game was addictive. I counted out the eighty cents for each collection to separate my earnings from Mr. Blake's. I put his money in my right pocket and my earnings in the left. Then I went Berzerk.

"Dammit," I said out loud to myself. I inserted another quarter. "I almost had the high score."

I dropped quarters until the left pocket emptied. It was time to go, but my right pocket was full of coins, begging for one more chance.

If I could get the high score, everyone would see the name Laney. "This business is built on trust," Mr. Blake had said. *I could always pay him next week.* "Intruder alert. Intruder alert," the android warned. I slid my hand into my right pocket and pulled out a quarter.

The next payday, Mr. Blake stared at the money on the table: just a few crinkled dollars and quarters.

"What happened?" Mr. Blake asked.

"People gave me rain checks," I said.

Monday morning, I showed up for my papers but they weren't there. How can you be a paper boy without papers? You can't.

Years later, it was discovered that Mr. Blake was "getting boys." Losing that paper route was a blessing.

Discarded.

Luther

While a kid in my sixth-grade class named Michael Fields read aloud the accomplishments of Booker T. Washington, I traced W. E. B. Du Bois's forehead in my history textbook—brother sure didn't have much hair. Neither did Mr. Garibel, who appeared in our doorway with his horseshoe hairline and clipboard.

"Please come with me if your name is called. Francisco Ramon, Carmen Arroyo, Deanna Moore…" Mr. Garibel said.

I gave no mind to the names called until I heard Deanna's name. Why was she being summoned with the geeks? I continued my tracing, ignoring the banal intrusion.

"And Rodney Laney," Mr. Garibel said.

I dropped my pencil and jumped at the opportunity to break free from the daily rut. We followed Mr. Garibel, the lead egghead, to a room just big enough to hold four desks.

"Since you guys excelled on the California Achievement Test, you've been selected to be in a math club."

He chalked enigmatic equations on the board, then helped us solve the problems he created. From then on, he randomly yanked us from class, which bugged Mrs. Nelson and delighted me.

Deanna became my first live model, whom I sketched without her noticing—a secondary skill I developed while learning high school algebra with Mr. Garibel. Capturing her high cheekbones, her most tantalizing trait, posed a challenge. I was distracted by her evocative lips, which were always yapping to other dudes.

Luther Vandross woke me up at 1 a.m. one day, telling me about the night he fell in love. I sat up in bed, listening to the lyrics sung by the lead singer of Change. The song ended, but the inspiration remained, and an idea was sparked.

In order to get the words, I needed to tape the song. I listened to the kitchen's radio cassette recorder for hours, with the red record and black play button depressed with my finger on the pause button. Stacks of songs played while I was under self-imposed house arrest. "Searchin'," one of Change's popular songs, played often, but it wasn't the one I was searching for. I mimicked the rooster on Looney Tunes, crooning to an imaginary Deanna.

I searched and sang in the kitchen, in the living room, and eventually in my bedroom. I grew impatient and recorded other love ballads, and although they didn't sway me, I found truth in them as well. Facedown on my pillow, I would nod off with my finger on the pause button. Somewhere in the night, the deejay finally spun my song. I released the pause button, then watched the reels capture my feelings.

The melody ended and the work began. I rewound and replayed the tape line by line. The tedious transcription lasted into early the next morning. After writing all the lyrics, I ended the page with two boxes: one for yes and one for no.

The next day was a Wednesday. I sat behind Deanna and waited, clutching Luther's words in my pocket. Perspiration from my palms dampened the letter and my spirits. The rooster had become a chicken. I negotiated with myself: *Thursday will be the day I give her the note.*

Thursday, I sat behind Deanna, still clutching Luther's words. *Friday. Friday will be the day.*

Friday came. Today would be the day I would inform Deanna about our relationship. Behind Deanna, I sat again, waiting for the moment when the other thirty students weren't watching, waiting for the moment she returned my smile, waiting for the moment to become "the night I fell in love."

The final bell rang. It was the weekend, and I was still waiting on the moment. My classmates donned their coats. I slipped into my goose-down leather jacket. Deanna put on her parka; her cheek-bones disappeared into her hood.

Freed from classroom eyes, Luther and I lagged behind Deanna. I knew if I didn't take a shot then, I wouldn't see her until the next week. My resolve quickened my pace. I tapped her shoulder. She turned. Deep in the tunnel of her hood was the face I had sketched so many times. I searched for the note but couldn't find it. Dammit.

Deanna waited with tunnel vision. "Deanna uh, um…would you, would you be my girl…friend?" I managed to get out. But my plan fell apart. A familiar expression came over Deanna's face. I recognized it from the time Mr. Garibel introduced her to quadratic equations. It was a look of utter bewilderment, but unlike that time in the classroom, she knew this answer.

"No."

That was the last note. I turned up the hill, dazed, on the coldest day in November, still searching.

Discarded.

Hoop Dreams

In late November, midway through sixth grade, basketballs pounded the hardwood in the musty air of the cafe-gym-atorium. (This was the nickname I gave the room since school twelve's cafeteria, gym, and auditorium were all the same space. Folding chairs and folding lunchroom tables made the difference.) Sweat flew off the players as they ran suicide drills. Their sneakers screeched as they dove to touch the red lines. With little ventilation, the gym was a hot crotch of drenched T-shirts. All of the jerseys were soaked, except for one belonging to one cold son of bitch.

I had never attempted to play organized b-ball before, or any sport for that matter. I knew I could compete since I always had to guard Eric, the most skilled of the fellas, in our pickup games. Nate Moore, my classmate and a born salesman, had sold me into trying out for school twelve's team with the lure of NBA fame and fortune. We rolled into tryouts, ready to give our best shots. Nate stepped onto the hardwood floor with hope; I stepped onto it with my FootJoys. My sneakers didn't matter because I was about to be tripped up by the school's disciplinarian: Dave.

My problem with Dave had started weeks before I entered the gym. During recess, someone had stolen money from Deanna, and to my surprise, she accused me. I use the term "money" loosely because it was a freakin' quarter.

Initially, I brushed off the accusations because of my crush, but the apple of my eye was rotten. That apple didn't fall far from a giant oak tree. Mr. Moore, a behemoth of a man who squeezed nickels and pinched pennies, was Deanna's dad. I had delivered papers to him, but when it came to collecting payment, it was old news every week.

"Come back next week," Mr. Moore would say. *You big broke-ass, seven-foot-thirteen, Green Giant–looking suckamother. You don't have a dollar and twenty cents?* I never said that to his face, but I had the courage to think it once I'd crossed the street.

Deanna intended to get me yoked up. She went to Dave, the paddle man, a security guard whose job description included doling out pain. Deanna leaned into his ear before pointing at me. He studied her for a heartbeat before laying eyes on me.

"He stole my quarter," Deanna said.

"No, I didn't," I exclaimed.

Dave slid his paddle to the side, then stuck his hand in his pocket and began probing. *Freakin' creep.* Then he pulled out a quarter and placed it in her hand. She raised the quarter; it sparkled in front of Dave's gold tooth. So enamored with the coin, Deanna didn't notice Dave slide his arm around her waist. My dismay turned into disdain.

Dave grabbed his paddle, then stared at me. In our neighborhood, it was said, "If you lie, then you steal." Thieves received unique scorn that came via contemptuous scowls. It was a look that I'd never seen until then. Dave opened his drawer and placed his paddle inside.

Nate shimmied out of his sweatpants, revealing his too-tight gym shorts as if there weren't enough balls in the gym already. I considered leaving. Out of all the faculty who could've been chosen to coach—Mr. Garibel, Mr. Howell, or even the maintenance man—why had they chosen the paddle man?

Dave sat on the stage eating chips. The chubby disciplinarian noticed me, snickered, then licked his fingers. He crushed the bag and chucked it in the trash. He cut me from the team the second he looked at me with that scowl. I knew it. He knew it. But he had to make it look good. He gave me a chance, albeit a fat one.

"We're going to play a three-on-three tournament. Rodney, if your team loses, you go home," Dave said. He picked all of his starters, including our school's star player, Kevin Williams, for one team. Then he fitted me with two other guys trying out. The other ballers crammed the sidelines. "First team to hit three buckets wins," Dave said.

Dave tossed the ball to his starters for the first takeout because they needed yet another advantage. Kevin took the inbound pass and sped up the court, pulled up at the corner, and took his shot. All net.

My team inbounded the ball and dished two chest passes before Kevin stole the third. He crossed his man over and drove up the court for an easy layup. Two-zip.

I took the inbound pass, dribbled up court, gave a head fake, stepped back, and hit a fadeaway jump shot. Swish. Two-one.

Kevin brought the ball up court. Our defense settled in. Big Clarence Presley on the starters team muscled his man back, hooking him with a violent elbow, which floored his defender and Dave—the latter due to laughter. A look-away pass from Kevin to a wide-open Clarence ended the game. I had scored against his starting squad; that had to mean something, right? Nope.

Dave used only his salty fingers to wave goodbye. It was a wave meant for a child. My million-dollar dream had been slain because of twenty-five cents.

Discarded.

Peanut

I had duped Mom into believing I received only one report card a year and that it came at random times. Whichever report card that ensured that an ass-whooping wouldn't follow was the one she received. "What about your sister, Tasha?" you might ask. "Didn't she receive a report card?" Bugs Bunny helped me get that under control.

I played a gag on Tasha that I'd seen on Looney Tunes. I stuck a match between her toes while she slept, lit it, then walked into the living room.

"Yeeeeeooooooowwwww!" she screamed.

Tasha burst into the living room with her hair going every which way. Smoke wafted from her big toe. Keeping a straight face proved impossible.

"I'm going to tell Mommy," she said.

She would've told Mom if Mom had been around, but by the time she came home, all was forgiven. Tasha couldn't stand to see me get beatings. It pained her as much as it did me.

I intercepted Tasha's report cards when mine were subpar. If she protested, all I had to do was strike a match. The warning kept her from ratting—that and the love for her big brother and her big toe.

Mom translated everything my teachers said into the language she understood. "Rodney didn't turn in his homework." *Whoop his ass.* "Rodney was late several times." *Whoop his ass.* "Rodney jokes too much." *Whoop his ass.* It had all started with my fifth-grade teacher in school twenty-eight, who winked as she told Mom that I was smarter than my grades reflected, and I just needed a little motivation. *Whoop his ass.*

Homework was the reason I lost so much ass in the sixth grade. Mrs. Nelson, an abrasive, militant woman, ruined my life by giving us so damn much of it.

Mrs. Nelson would hand out warning notices in an envelope. "Don't open the envelope. Give it to your parents, have them sign it, and return it tomorrow." *Yeah, right.* As soon as I crossed the street, I read the notice, and it read "Whoop his ass."

To preserve my hide, I decided to sign it myself. I found an old report card and notes to study Mom's penmanship. I traced her John Hancock several times before writing it on the dotted line. I handed it to Mrs. Nelson as if I was feeding raw meat to a tiger. She casually filed it away with the other notices. Thus starting my trials in forgery.

Every time Mrs. Nelson sent home a derogatory notice, I penned Mom's name on the dotted line. My derriere rejoiced in the preservation.

One evening, after Mom slid a plate in front of Freddy, she pulled a letter from the wooden mail caddy attached to the wall.

"I thought it was tonight. Get ready," she said.

"Where we going?"

"To this parent-teacher thing they having tonight."

Oh shit!

"For real?" I said.

How the hell did that slip by me? Tasha.

"Let's go," Mom said.

Mrs. Nelson explained to Mom that my grades could be better if I applied myself. (Ass-whooping.) "I sure wish I would've been notified about this earlier," Mom said. Mrs. Nelson, taken aback, showed Mom *all* the warning notices she "had signed." "I didn't sign those," Mom said.

If I pass out right now and go to the hospital...

Mom gave Mrs. Nelson permission to discipline me whenever she saw fit. They shook hands, united in the battle to make me a better student. Do I even have to say what happened that night?

"Rodney, if you don't bring your homework in tomorrow, I'm going to light yo ass up," Mrs. Nelson warned. No problem.

Nothing in the December sky the next morning suggested the day would be extraordinary. Keith and I rushed to school to beat the bell. Half a block away from the school, minutes before the late bell, a memory flashed: "I'm going to light yo ass up." I froze.

I'd forgotten to do my damn homework. With Mom's blessing, Mrs. Nelson would keep her promise. Keith searched my face for an explanation for the sudden stop. Mentally, I built my case for why Keith should accompany me. I prepared for the serious persuasion and the candy bribes.

"Keith, let's cut school," I finally said.

"OK."

Damn, that was easy. We about-faced, and for the first time, we played hooky. The morning discord—the diesel engines, the blaring music, and the lively crowds—all faded with each wandering step. The empty streets left Keith and me exposed as the temperature plummeted. I blew steamy breaths into my cupped hands, then stuck them deep into my pockets, reaching for any warmth. Keith's frail body trembled, and his chattering teeth drew my attention.

"We have to watch for truant officers," I said.

"What's that?"

"Men who shoot kids for skipping school."

"Nah, you lying."

We wandered northwest into Prospect Park, a predominantly white borough, where all the snowmen pointed at us. Christmas decorations adorned the windows. Keith wrestled himself, battling the bitterness. I needed to find us a warm place to chill and relieve his misery.

We came upon a golden bull as if we were in a damn fable. The bull's metallic muscles gleamed as it guarded the door, which I noticed was ajar. The Golden Steer restaurant appeared closed to customers. We slipped past the bull and snuck into the bathroom.

Fresh ammonia nuked our noses as we slid across the slippery floor. I ran warm water over my hands and felt the heat in my ankles. Keith thawed and bathed in the warmth, and his teeth slowly came back under his control. I was planning to stay there for as long as possible.

A white man wheeled in a mop bucket. He jumped back, startled.

"What y'all doing in here?" he asked us.

"Using the bathroom," I said.

"Get out of here before I call the police."

After a short time back outdoors, Keith's teeth were chattering again. I looked at my watch. It read 9:50. Damn, it wasn't even 10 a.m.

"I can't feel my toes. I think I'm getting frostbite," Keith said.

He wasn't going to make it.

"Let's go to school," Keith said.

Go to school late and without my homework? Mrs. Nelson would murder me.

"I'll find us a spot," I said.

I led us uphill, back toward Paterson. A narc's car drove by, making me turn my face away. The constant rubbing of my hands and blowing lukewarm breath into them didn't give any relief. I needed to use my noggin, or as Freddy would say, my peanut. Peanut? A light pierced my fog. "I got the perfect spot, Keith."

At the back of a three-story house, I opened the basement window and pulled myself through, then extended a hand to Keith. Our homeboy Peanut lived on the second floor and had shown us how to access his basement. At the time, it seemed like information I would never need. I wondered what would be his next lesson: how to get into the safe? Peanut was living up to his name.

We stumbled through the darkness, knocking over boxes and dusty furnishings, making certain our "silent" break-in could be heard by anyone within earshot. Footsteps descended the staircase on the other side of the wall, then stopped. I halted Keith with a finger to my lips. Be quiet. We listened.

The footsteps retreated; we were safe. I discovered a back room with boxes stacked to the ceiling. Keith found a cubbyhole and nestled in. I scaled a set of boxes, then lay over them and drifted off.

A beam of light awakened me. It scanned the front room. Its source: a looming, dark figure. An icy draft swirled into the room, where Keith and I remained motionless.

The beam swept right to left until it entered our room. It didn't spot us at first. I turned my head, ensuring I would be face to face with whoever was holding the flashlight.

The man jumped back, reaching for his gun.

"Get yo ass down from there!"

"Both of us?" I asked.

"Who else in here?" the man asked.

He whipped his flashlight between two boxes, revealing Keith's scowl. Two suited men escorted us to their squad car, their walkie-talkies chirping. The narc car smelled stale and criminal. The front seat pressed against my knees, making me squirm. The detective radioed in a call about a break-in. *A break-in? Who broke-in?* I wondered.

"Where do y'all live?" the policeman asked.

"Right there," Keith said.

Keith pointed at our apartment complex.

"Is your mother home?"

"Mine's not," I said.

"If your mothers aren't home, I'm going to have to take y'all downtown," he said.

My heart flickered as I recalled when Uncle Kenny had warned us about narcs taking people downtown: "You better hope they take you downtown and not Moosey Lot." Moosey Lot was where some cops executed their own justice. "My mom's home," Keith said, tears drizzling into his lap. I rested my roasting peanut of a head against the cold glass of the car window.

The detective rang my doorbell even though I'd told him Mom was working. I was relieved when she didn't answer. I'd rather have taken my chances in Moosey Lot. The knock on Ms. Carol's door resounded in the tiny vestibule. I was certain old nosey Mrs. Smith, the neighborhood herald, who lived on the first floor, would pop her head into the hallway to investigate. Keith inclined his head toward the door. The detective sighed and banged again. Nothing. He radioed to his partner: "No answer." He motioned us with his walkie-talkie to return to the car. We were headed downtown. Keith looked up at me, lips trembling. I saw all my fault in his eyes.

Then Ms. Carol's door swung open, and she took charge. "I'll teach you to break into people's basements," Ms. Carol said. News in the hood traveled fast. "Get yo ass upstairs," she said. The detective left me in the custody of Ms. Carol, a woman known for her unorthodox style of punishment we called the Nestle plunge.

According to Mrs. Smith, Ms. Carol would line Keith or Jaima at the top of their staircase, facing her with their backs to the steps. She would chant, "Get ready. Get ready. Get ready. 'Cause Imma whoop yo ass." Then she would push them.

I resolved that if she tried pushing me down those stairs, she was coming with me. I sat in their living room, listening to Keith's screams from the bedroom as Ms. Carol tore into him. "Don't think you're getting away with this shit, Rodney," Ms. Carol shouted at me too.

My peanut was on fire, searching for a story; cutting school for failing to do homework wouldn't keep the skin on my back. A knock at the door paused the cracking of the belt. Ms. Carol stormed from the bedroom, then scampered down the stairs. Then I heard Mom's voice.

"Yeah, he here," Ms. Carol said.

She returned to the top of the steps. I gripped the railing as I walked past her. Each descending step revealed more of Mom until I could see her gritted teeth and furrowed brow. I slinked by her, expecting a whack to the back of my head. At our door, she said: "Get in there and take them clothes off."

I fumbled with each button on my shirt. Mom slammed her keys on the kitchen table and peeled off her coat. "That cop said he could've shot you."

Her interpretation: make certain I would never again be in a situation where a cop would feel threatened enough to shoot me. She pulled out an extension cord, doubled it, then quadrupled it. The lash hung at her side, cocked and loaded. Mom began firing.

When it was over, I lay on my bed, knowing how Jesus felt. Mom had taken off work to go Christmas shopping. She'd been in the bank across the street when the security guard told her the police had a kid in custody who resembled me. She assured him that her son was in school and couldn't possibly be in the back of a police car. But he was wearing a uniform, so she obliged him.

"You're not getting anything for Christmas," Mom said.

The next day, I hung my coat on one of the classroom hooks and eased my sore ass into my desk chair. I readied myself for the day's lesson.

"Rodney, where's your homework?" Mrs. Nelson asked.

Oh shit. Mrs. Nelson pulled her belt from her drawer.

"I warned you," she said.

Discarded.

Boy Scouts

One day while I was choking the shit out of Eric, a good Samaritan broke up our fight. After filling his lungs with the air he'd been deprived of for thirty or forty seconds, Eric punched me in the jaw, then scurried up the stairs. I glared at Eric's savior.

"That's why I was choking him," I told him.

"Take it easy, son," he said.

I rubbed my jaw and contemplated kicking the meddler in the shin.

"Take a look at this," he said.

He stuck a pamphlet in my hand—as if I was in the mood to read some shit. I rolled my lower jaw and hiked up the steps. "It will do you some good," he shouted.

Boy Scouts of America? The only thing I knew about the Boy Scouts was that they rubbed sticks to make fire, a skill about as useful as a used toothpick. Pictured on the brochure were white boys in whack uniforms, camping and looking all gleeful. A scout pulled a bow, aiming an arrow at an unforeseen target—perhaps his sixth-grade teacher. The meetings were at Gilmore Memorial Tabernacle church, three blocks down the hill. I showed the brochure to Mom, and she studied it for a minute. "I wonder when you'll get a uniform," she said.

Keith's eagerness to join with me didn't surprise me, but Ms. Carol's enthusiasm did. "That sounds motherfuckin' wholesome," she said.

We attended a 6 p.m. meeting at Gilmore. Fifteen or so boys filled the pews, ranging in age from seven to fifteen, all waiting for *the man*. The few adults in the room cheered when famed local track star Franklin Jacobs walked to the podium. He preached about camping trips and survival skills. Keith and I fist-bumped, amped for the chance to experience nature outside of Paterson. All that Mr. Jacobs required from us was weekly attendance and weekly $10 dues.

I toted my Boy Scout handbook in one hand and icy ammunition in the other the next time we headed to the church for a meeting. The darkening sky was our only cover. The virtues of being a good Boy Scout hadn't sunk in yet, and Franklin Jacobs had forgotten to preach, "Thou shalt not pelt passing cars with snowballs." Keith tossed his tiny balls while I gunned mine. We usually hid behind the bushes atop the stairs when targeting buses, vans, and jalopies, but we had somewhere else to be on this frosty evening.

Less than a block away from the church, my spidey-sense started tingling. A grim-looking person marched in our direction, igniting my fight-or-flight mechanism. I spun off, leaving behind tracks and a bewildered Keith. The blur took off after me. My high stepping would've made Franklin Jacobs proud. I ran up the hill and darted through the alleyway leading toward Peanut's backyard. Keys jingled, alerting me of my follower's proximity.

The wooden staircase creaked as I leaped up two, three, four stairs at a time. No way he could catch me in my hood. Plus, I had a plan. I waited for him to ascend the staircase. I knew exactly what I had to do.

Once he ran up the stairs, I jumped from the second floor, then ran back up the alleyway we had taken seconds before. Ha ha, sucker! I crossed Haledon Avenue toward the bank parking lot, headed away from home. Then *jingle jingle.*

Damn. I hopped a fence, landed on Hopper Street, then headed toward a house on the corner of Inglis Street. Thick bushes ran alongside the house, making it a good hiding spot—I hoped.

Jingle. Jingle.

His steel-toed boots and khaki pants slowed as he came up to the bushes. He took the deep breaths my lungs were screaming for. He knew I was in the bushes. Branches cracked and twigs popped as the leaves parted between his fingers, then snapped back after his release. He took a step closer, repeating the process. The cracking and snapping grew louder.

If my labored breathing didn't give away my position, my pounding heartbeat would. I sprang like a jackrabbit from the bushes and tore down the street toward school twelve. I turned left at the school, then headed down the hill, gasping.

My energy and will were depleted by the time I reached the bottom. I bent over, exhausted, desperate for air. I couldn't run anymore. All I could do was watch as the maniac closed in.

He was the wrong mafucka to have thrown a snowball at. You know how I found out? Because he kept telling me. "You messed with the wrong mafucka!" He jerked me back and forth periodically, stopping to ask: "You know who you messed with?"

Hmmm, I believe I know this one.

"The wrong mafucka."

I agree.

"That's right. Today you messed with the wrong mafucka."

The geezer held me by the nape of my neck until we reached Roger's. He pushed open the door. Barbara looked up from behind the register. Now everyone would know. I started doing damage control. "The phone is in the back, Dad," I said.

I have no idea why I said that. The man gave me so much attention, I'd made him a father figure. My "dad" called the police, and we waited in a dysfunctional silence. When the police arrived, pops reported that his car had been struck by a snowball. I said it wasn't me, it was the other guy. (Don't judge me; Keith wasn't around.)

Mr. Marathon admitted he didn't see who threw the snowball and the reason he'd chased me was that I ran. The policeman asked me why I ran.

"Because he was chasing me," I said.

"Is there any damage?" the policeman asked. The man shook his head no, then left.

"Where do you live?" the policeman asked me.

"Up the street."

He opened the back door of his cruiser, and I crammed myself into the cage, where the seats didn't give a damn and the smell was awfully familiar. Roger's patrons peered at the police cruiser. My hood prevented them from seeing my face—I made sure of it.

A metal partition separated me from the officer. He snapped on the bubble light, whipped a U-turn, drove two blocks, hooked another U-turn, and double-parked. He opened my door and I scooted out, holding my *Boy Scout Handbook*. While we waited for Mom to answer the door, he asked to see my book.

"Are you a scout?" he asked.

"Yes, sir."

Mom opened the door to see her son with a tall white police officer. She needed a cigarette immediately.

"Good evening, ma'am," he said to her. "Is this your son?"

He detailed both stories, mine and the wrong mafucka's. My version was: It wasn't me. Mom scoured my face, searching for any sign of a lie. She looked to the officer. "Do you believe him?"

The policeman eyed me, then my handbook. "I do," he said. With those two words, he saved my ass.

At the next Boy Scouts meeting, we learned how fast Franklin Jacobs really was when he ran off with our money. Keith and I never learned how to make a fire, but we learned how to get burned. If the Boy Scouts would've lasted, maybe, just maybe, that would've been my last run-in with the police.

Discarded.

The Dirty South

One day just after sixth grade was over, Keith stood in our doorway under my armpit watching Mom, who was hustling in the kitchen.

"Where y'all going?" Keith asked.

"Down South," I said.

"Oh, OK. When you coming back?"

"I don't know."

The locals never questioned what "down South" meant. The vague term only prompted more questions from teachers and other outsiders. For us, "down South" meant Lancaster, South Carolina.

"Who's all going with y'all?" Keith asked.

"It's us and Aunt Mildred and them," I said.

Mom filled a cooler with sandwiches, fried chicken, potato salad, and no-frills sodas. She stashed dozens of boxes of Nabisco cookies into a brown bag she was planning to give to her brothers and sister.

The smell of the chicken opened Keith's nostrils. He licked his ashy lips, dropping a hint. *That food is for the road trip, buddy.* Mom packed enough food to feed us, Aunt Mildred's carload, and everyone else on I-95.

I hid my excitement, knowing Keith wouldn't be leaving the city for the summer. He wanted to come with us, but we both knew Ms.

Carol wouldn't allow it. It wasn't a question of room. The back seat of Freddy's car was the size of a twin bed. The real reason was that he wasn't family, and being blood brothers didn't count.

I didn't want to rush Keith off since I knew I wasn't going to be seeing him for a week or so, but I had to finish packing. "Alright, homey, I gotta go," I said. I gave him a pound and closed the door.

Visiting historical places such as Mount Rushmore or the Lincoln Memorial during our summer vacations wasn't an option. The only monument we got to see otherwise was Pedro, the one-hundred-foot-tall mascot at the South of the Border tourist attraction. And the only history we were used to seeing was our own.

In the fields we saw on our drive down South, the cows chewed as if they were going to blow bubbles. Birds that looked just like Heckle and Jeckle from the cartoon perched on a bundle of hay. The cotton fields returned Mom to her hay days.

"We used to have to get up every morning at five a.m. and pick cotton before school—when we was allowed to go to school," Mom said.

I imagined how it must've been, being raised in a small home with fourteen other bodies coming and going, bumping or brushing against someone or something at every turn from breakfast to dinner. With so many kids, they must've been starving all the time.

"Did you guys ever go hungry?" I asked.

"Never. We grew our own vegetables and picked enough to be canned. Deddie made us pick enough to sell."

Well, that's refreshing, I thought.

"Deddie use to hire us out to a white man after we picked enough for him."

Well, that's unrefreshing.

"The only time we got a day off from the fields was when it rained or in the wintertime after the harvest."

I knew her standard button was coming.

"You guys don't know how good you got it," she said.

I imagined Mom's fingers pulling the cotton from the stalks, with her being careful not to prick a finger. I imagined her father as an overseer, cracking the belt when my uncles were horseplaying. I imagine my uncle Larry and uncle Gucci tired and brooding, staring at that strap. I imagine in those fields is where Deddie's demise was conceived.

Freddy pulled the Bonneville off the paved road. Dust clouds kicked up behind us as the Michelin tires crunched along the dirt road. The bumpiness swayed the taut plastic shopping bag stuffed with chicken bones and empty soda cans. Hens scattered as the car came to a stop in front of the McNeals' residence. They had a real barn with a real tractor and real hogs. We were staying with Mom's younger sister, Aunt Mern, and her family, while Aunt Mildred and Eddie would be staying with Uncle Herald.

When we drove up, the curtains jostled before the screen door swung open, and cousins Brendan, Tymeka, and Jewettee spilled onto the porch with buttermilk smiles. After a round of hugs, the screen door cracked shut with the aunts and uncles on the inside and the cousins on the outside.

The McNeals' house was where Mom had grown up. The family lost everything when Mom's first childhood home burned down. A new house was built, and Aunt Mern inherited it.

I breathed in the surroundings. The neighboring house was a tractor-trailer minus the tractor. The Traps, their other neighbors, lived down the road, round the bend, in the woods. I took their word for it.

Chris and Shawn, my uncle Herald's kids, were en route, according to Brendan.

"What do y'all do for fun?" I asked Brendan.

He contemplated.

"Run," he said.

"Run just to run," I scoffed. "Where I'm from, we run with a purpose." We ran to catch the ice cream truck, to play tag, or to avoid molestation.

Eddie instigated a footrace between Brendan and me. While I stood a foot taller than my younger cousin, it was the days of hauling ass that really stoked my confidence. I was a shoo-in.

Tymeka jogged down the road, stopping even with the barn. She twirled around, making her pigtails swivel, and extended her arms, creating a Jesus-like finish line. I took my mark. Brendan focused on Jesus.

"On your mark. Get set. Go!" Eddie said.

Brendan ran as if that was all he ever did. Because it was. Without a brute behind me, I couldn't run as fast as I thought. Brendan's chest stayed at my shoulder until we reached Tymeka. Thanks to my long arms, I pulled out the win.

"Let's go again," Brendan said.

"No problem."

My neck and chest were glazed with sweat. Brendan wasn't even perspiring. We walked back to Eddie, who was chucking rocks into the cornfield.

"Brendan almost got you," Eddie said.

The next race wouldn't be close, I promised. I took my mark.

"Hold on a second," Brendan said. He kicked off his sneakers.

He about to run barefoot? He was pulling a Fred Flintstone. I gaped at his toes and at his heels, which could cut glass.

Eddie raised his hand over his head, grinning crookedly for a second, then he yanked his hand down, shouting "Go!"

Neck and neck, we chopped down the dirt road headed straight to salvation. Brendan eked out a lead, kicking up dust with his toes, running past Jesus and never looking back. I kept my promise. It wasn't close.

That night, the darkness washed away the South Carolina heat. I clapped my sneakers together to remove the gunk. I was covered in stank and couldn't wait to scrub off the country crud from my crevices, but that's when things really got funky.

"After you finish washing, don't let the water out. You guys are going to use the same water," Aunt Mern said.

Wait. What?

I questioned Aunt Mern using my "inside voice." Sometimes you know when you're going to get an ass-whooping. After that ridiculously foul news, I knew. No way was I going to bathe in the same sweaty, all-day-running-around-in-the-pasture funky-ass bathwater that my cousins used. Even the hogs were thinking, *She can't be serious.* The only way I would go along with that plan was if I got to wash up first.

"Let the young ladies go first," Aunt Mern said. *Dammit.*

When it was my turn, I sat my clean white towel on the toilet and stared at the mud. I remembered the time Mom had whipped me while I was in the tub when that leather had cracked against my wet ass and spread webs of pain up my back and made me do the Electric Boogie. I examined the debris floating in the fecal-looking wash. *You gotta be outta your goddamn mind if you think I'm going to bathe in that shit.*

I locked the door and drained the tub. I opened the tap halfway for fresh water and shut it off every time I heard footsteps, slowly filling the tub enough to wash in. I sunk one foot into the water; it was cold but clean. I scrubbed every nook and cranny twice, needing to soil the water to avoid suspicion. My heart went out to the next bather.

I dried off and slipped into my PJs, mission accomplished. I opened the bathroom door to where Aunt Mern was standing.

"You finished?" she asked.

"Yeah. I mean yes, ma'am."

She observed the bathwater and raised an eyebrow. "Did you run new bathwater?"

I stalled and feigned stupidity. *Did she know? If she told Mom, I'd be doing the Electric Boogie again. Aunt Mern will believe whatever I say since she has no reason to think I would lie to her.* "Yes, ma'am," I admitted.

The water appeared scummy enough to me, but I guessed it wasn't. I tensed up, bracing myself for the scalding.

"OK," Aunt Mern said. That was it? No punishment or scolding? That's when Aunt Mern became my favorite auntie.

The next morning, fresh bacon crackled in the skillet and the smell of Aunt Mern's baked biscuits filled the kitchen when she opened the oven. Mom set the table. I lingered in case they needed a taster. "You're going to have to wait, Rodney," Mom said. She knew what I wanted. Aunt Mern's biscuits were legendary, and so was the number of them I could devour. "Rodney, tell your cousins to come inside," Aunt Mern said.

Uncle Herald's and Aunt Mildred's car pulled into the front yard just as I hollered. "Come and get it." The only people who could hear me were family. It filled me with pride. I shouted again. "Come and get it!" From the porch, I let everyone know it was time to break bread.

On the table sat a pile of golden-brown biscuits, finally within reaching distance. We assembled around the table, waiting for Uncle Doug, Aunt Marion's husband, who was in the bathroom. Mom fixed my plate and sat the saucer of biscuits under my nose. The butter slid off the flaky crust into my saucer of molasses. My mouth filled with pining juice. When Uncle Doug joined us, we all clasped hands. "Let's bow our heads," Uncle Doug said. He blessed the food, giving the family permission to dig into the grub.

In the McNeals' living room, a photo of a fair-skinned Native American-looking woman highlighted the console table. I had seen only one picture of my grandmother alone. I admired her likeness in the aged photo. She was in her twenties, I guessed.

"You grandmomma was a beautiful woman, wasn't she?" Aunt Mildred said. Mom and my aunts' tone was tender whenever they spoke of my grandmother Marion. I wondered why Aunt Mern, whose name was short for Marion, had received Grandma's name.

Another photo of Grandma with Grandad was more common. I held it up to see: Jesse Belle, a dark and serious man, looked as if he never heard a joke, or at least not a good one. Uncle Gucci favored him. On her way out for her after-meal cigarette, Mom paused.

"That's the Laney scowl, you see," Mom said.

"What's that?" I said.

She pursed her lips, showing a sliver of teeth. It was a look I'd seen many times before, usually right before an ass-whooping. I just didn't know it had a name.

"Your granddaddy kept her pregnant," Aunt Mildred said. I knew the story, but Aunt Mildred was going to tell it again. "They married when Ma was fifteen, 'cause she was pregnant. Um-hmm. A condition she'd be in for the next twenty-two years...."

I put the picture back on the bureau and inched toward the door.

"She popped out Lucy, J. B., uhh…Herl, Margie, Kitty, Luberta, me, then there was…uh, Mern, Larry, Gucci, Scott, Teresa—she was stillborn, but she still counts—and Vicky. Um-hmm, all by the age of thirty-seven," Aunt Mildred said.

Damn.

"The only alone time I had with my momma was when she was doing my hair," Mom said. A heaviness sunk in my stomach deeper than the biscuits when she said that.

Aunt Mern finished cleaning up the kitchen. "Rodney, I saved a couple of biscuits if you want some more," she said. Maybe that's the reason she had Grandma's name. So I could pretend she was Grandma when she laughed; so I could pretend she was Grandma when we hugged; so I could pretend I knew what it meant to have a grandma.

My uncles rarely spoke of grandma unless provoked. It seemed that much of the family history had been blotted out. I headed outside toward the dark spot in my family's history. A well in the middle of the yard touched the long shadow cast by the barn. The decaying wood and hay temporarily smothered the smell of the swine. A massive tractor stood in the dark spot with its back to us as if it had something to hide. Its rusted tire came up to my chest. It filled one side of the barn, the barn in which the Laneys' lives had been forever altered. More than one of my uncles had been in the barn the day Grandad was murdered. More than one of my uncles had pointed a gun at him, but only one uncle took the blame and served the time.

Perhaps it was in our DNA. Or perhaps we were just hardheaded. Whatever the reason, Eddie and I were bound to get the switch at some point that summer. Eddie's luck ran out first. Aunt Mildred sent him to get his own switch. What kind of psychological mind fart was that? Of course, Eddie brought back a twig. He hoped it would soften his punishment. It did not. It only infuriated Aunt Mildred. He tried to switch the switch, but it was too late. Aunt Mildred uprooted a small pecan tree and planted it on his ass.

My luck didn't last long either. Whatever I said or did, I don't remember. What followed eclipsed the inconsequential details. What I do remember is getting summoned to the house by an irate Mom. "Oooh, you gonna get it," Brendan said.

No big deal, I pretended. I whistled as I strolled into the house. The whistling promptly turned into screaming. All my family members heard the pain. All my cousins knew the feeling.

When I went back outside, darkness had fallen over the front yard, the well, and the barn.

Discarded.

Noodle

As the elevator doors closed, I knew something was wrong. I stood behind a custodian dressed in a white uniform. I didn't want to see his face. And I didn't want him seeing mine. He uncoiled his keychain, searching for a key. He stopped once he found the one shaped like a hollow bullet. He inserted it into a keyhole at the top of a panel, then pressed the isolated button below it.

When we reached our floor, our escort gestured for us to exit. I followed Aunt Mildred and Mom onto the guarded floor. The smell of Pine-Sol attacked us as we stepped into the psych ward of Bergen Pines. Mom accompanied Aunt Mildred as she spoke with the medical personnel. Eddie walked up.

"Let me show you around," he said.

I'd been expecting a giant Native American, shaved heads, and padded walls like I'd seen in *One Flew Over the Cuckoo's Nest*, but I saw only a grown man sucking his thumb and a woman talking to herself—shit you see in downtown Paterson daily. I looked for some of my grammar school teachers.

"See the chick over there?" Eddie asked.

"The one drooling in the corner?"

"Yeah. I banged her."

Eddie pointed out another chick he'd finger-blasted, piquing my interest. I took a second look at the driveling diva. "What do I have to do to get in here?" I asked him.

Eddie's big-hearted laugh lifted my spirit. At that moment, we could've been anywhere. The reason he had been admitted to the hospital never came up.

"You know when you coming home?" I asked.

Eddie shrugged his shoulders. I couldn't tell if he wanted to or not. Mom and Aunt Mildred followed a white coat toward us. By the looks on their faces, the news wasn't good.

Would this be the last time I would see him in the psych ward? I'd pondered the same question later when we left the psych wards at Barnert Hospital, St. Joseph's, and Greystone too. I'd never seen Eddie "wild out." After leaving the ward one day, I asked Mom if she knew what was going on with him. She sighed and shook her head no. I went into Encyclopedia Brown mode and began theorizing.

I remembered one time when Eddie had been sitting across from me in his kitchen staring at his plate of soggy noodles. I chomped another bite of the delicious spaghetti—at least I'd psyched myself up to believe it was delicious. Wasting food was a crime in our family, but wasting Aunt Mildred's food was a capital offense.

Eddie pushed the trash aside and scraped his noodles into the bottom of the garbage bin, where they would feel at home. He covered them with rubbish to hide the evidence and pointed to his temple, indicating he was smart. I gave him a thumbs-up and considered a similar course of action until Aunt Mildred entered the kitchen with intent. She glanced at Eddie's plate.

"You think you slick, huh?" she said.

Guided by a mom's intuition, she started rummaging through the muck in the bin. She grabbed his plate and fork and started scooping up the spaghetti from the trash. She found each noodle, slopping them down on his plate.

"When I say eat your food, I mean it," she told him.

My jaw dropped. Then I quickly filled it with a gob of noodles. I kept my head down, twirling another spindle of spaghetti. Aunt Mildred slammed the plate in front of Eddie.

"Eat it," she ordered.

While Eddie dug into his tainted noodles, I added fresh pepper and a new perspective to mine. Best damn spaghetti I ever ate.

Back in the psych ward, Encyclopedia Brown surmised it was that type of stuff that could make anyone crack.

Discarded.

Blindsided

I damn near broke the hinges on the door when I slammed it shut, causing snow to fall like an avalanche from the roof. At thirteen, I'd grown taller than Mom, and to maintain her dominance, she'd put extra heat on the whip. And to rub hot sauce in the wound, she made me go to the store afterward. Anger consumed me, growing in my chest, the kind of rage that the freezing temperature couldn't thaw.

The snow buried everything immovable. Blackened slush splashed my boots, kicked off the tires of an asshole driving a rusty Trans Am. The heavy snow was ideal for making beefy snowballs. If the dick hadn't sped off, I would've pelted his window. I got whatever Mom forced me to buy, then trudged back uphill. As I neared the steps of our complex, a cold whack to my forehead stunned me. Snow oozed down my forehead as an uproar of laughter seeped into my awareness as I regained my balance. The bushes had sheltered the attack by the fellas, who were rejoicing in their successful strike. But I was the wrong motherfucka that day.

I ran up to the stairs looking for payback. "Who did it?" They all pointed at Kenny.

Before I tell you what happened, here's a little background on the guy who is about to be on the receiving end of my fury.

Kenny's mom, a solid, intimidating woman, didn't take smack from anyone. She treated Kenny and his brother like royalty. Kept them stocked with the newest gizmos and hippest fashions. You'd expect nothing less from a woman named Queenie. She strove to shelter her babies and keep them seen in the best light, but in our hood, sometimes lights got extinguished, and the best intentions were often blindsided.

Kenny couldn't have known the state that I was in. Hell, I couldn't have known what I was capable of. If I had, I would've walked away, but I threw punches instead, unleashing a rage with no regard for his defense. The punches landed on Kenny, but I was punching something else.

Kenny laid facedown on a sloped concrete embankment. The clamor from the fellas pierced my haze. Slosh fell from the raised boot I held over the back of Kenny's head. The craze should've been finished, but it wasn't. I stomped the back of his head. Then it was over. The ruckus died.

I dropped Mom's shit on the kitchen table, then went to my room. I sat on the edge of my bed and buried my forehead into my palms as the feeling of anger gave way to anxiety. What had I done?

Outside my window, I heard Ms. Queenie receive the news. *It wouldn't be long now.* The doorbell went crazy. "Valerie, open the door," yelled Ms. Queenie. Valerie was my mom's first name, but her friends called her Kitty.

I went into the living room to look out the window. Mom tied her housecoat belt around her waist, rushing to the door while looking at me.

"What the hell is going on out there?" she asked me.

I said nothing. She opened the door.

"Look at what Rodney did to my son's face," Ms. Queenie fumed. Kenny hung behind his mom. Glasses crushed. Face bloodied. Mom turned to me for an explanation.

"He hit me in the face with a snowball," I said.

"It wasn't me," Kenny said.

"Yes, you did!"

"No, I didn't."

"Go to your room," Mom ordered me.

The commotion moved from our porch past my window. The front door shut. *It wouldn't be long now.* I expected another round with a tougher opponent.

My mom came into my room. "You OK?" she asked.

I nodded.

"Dinner will be ready in a few," she said.

I didn't give much thought to Mom's empathy because a knuckle in my right hand absorbed my attention. I held my hand up to the light to see the damage. It truly was something else.

Discarded.

Straight Street

I was too young to work legally. Uncle Butch, a well-known police officer in our neighborhood, used his connections to get Eddie and me a weekends-only summer job at the Straight Street car wash. We worked twelve-hour shifts from 7 a.m. to 7 p.m. for twenty bucks plus tips.

Four heavy garage doors opened the concrete building to daylight and the Straight Street traffic. Adjacent to the car wash sat a small used-car lot packed with dusty vehicles. Smudged cars would line up from the car wash entrance back to the traffic light. When the cars exited the bay, they were as clean as pinto beans.

My station was to the left of the exit, behind a four-foot wall that extended from the building. I was in charge of drying towels. Every morning, I would drag thick wooden skids from their piles about thirty yards toward two steel barrels; I'd have to break them apart to use them as firewood. Some skids were flimsy and broke apart with little effort; most were not. Using my bare hands would earn me several splinters. When yanking with my arms wasn't enough to break off a board, I resorted to my Shaolin-style kung fu kicks.

The sun and the flames burned away any shadows. Sweat would sop my T-shirt and blue wave cap. I kept the fires burning in those steel barrels near the clothesline to dry the towels. Each time I dumped in new wood, the blaze would kick up, filling the air and my lungs with smoke.

The old dudes washed the cars while the young bucks dried. "Bossman," the owner, sloshed his rag with as much vigor as his employees. Where the suds ended and his white beard began was indeterminable. His partner, "G-man," talked incessantly—either to himself or to Bossman. I couldn't be sure since Bossman never acknowledged him.

"Grayman" was older than both of them and probably every-one else on the planet. His hunched back gave him the perfect posture for vacuuming cars. "Slim" kept a pint of gin in his shirt pocket, waiting for the clock to strike twelve. That's when Bossman allowed sipping.

Even the younger guys gulped at noon—mainly Olde English or Private Stock malt liquor, or gin. Supposedly, the young guys' drinking was unacceptable. Not because some of them were under-age, but because they were *righteous*.

They were members of the Nation of Gods and Earths—the Nation for short, also known as the Five Percenters. Being a mem-ber, or "being down" with the Nation, meant you were held to a higher standard. Was it a religion, a cult, or a gang? I couldn't tell.

The Nation of Gods and Earths started in New York, most likely Harlem. It hit Paterson as hard and as fast as crack would. It was built on the principle that 10 percent of the world knew the truth of existence and kept it from eighty-five percent of the world, thus keeping them ignorant. The Five Percenters knew the truth and supposedly were going to teach it to people like me: the ignorant.

"New Jeru," short for New Jerusalem, became Paterson's new nickname. The Nation taught that the original people, collectively known as the Asiatic Blackman, were God. Hip-hop culture helped the movement spread, with many of the popular rappers, such as Rakim, Big Daddy Kane, and King Sun, becoming members. It was a fad for many who only wanted to wear the garb, the necklaces, and the motherland pendant. The pendant, the symbol of the movement, was a star with a "7" in the center for Africa, that swung from the inflated chests of young Black men throughout New Jeru.

In order to be righteous, you had to follow the rules, which made it honorable. Members couldn't eat swine or drink alcohol and had to comprehend and memorize the "Supreme Mathematics." If they didn't, there were consequences. If Five Percenters ran into someone claiming to be righteous, they would form a circle—called the cipher—and a challenge would start by one of them saying: "What's the day's degree?" Or "What's today's mathematics?" A typical reply might have been:

"Today's mathematics is wisdom, knowledge, all being born to understanding. The primary objective of today's reality is to act only upon that which is known to be right and exact...."

The discussion about mathematics would've left my old teacher Mr. Garibel scratching his bald spot. If the supposedly righteous person made a mistake in their response, another type of lesson came in the form of a universal beatdown.

Their most inflammatory belief was that the white man was the devil. *Wait a minute*, I thought. *You mean to tell me Mr. Garibel is the devil? He doesn't have hair or horns on his head."* That meant the Six-Million Dollar Man was Lucifer? What about Mr. Rogers? No way, José. It was harder to defend Evel Knievel.

The righteous had to change their names. According to the beliefs of the Nation, the names given to them were government names, as if Uncle Sam had been in the delivery room with a clipboard: "We'll call this one Ray Ray. This one Tanique with a 'Q.' Here's a Shaquetta if I ever saw one."

Five Percenters took their new names seriously. Calling one of them by their government name was taken as disrespect and warranted a jab to the chest or worse. They chose supernatural names such as Universal Mathematics, Supreme God Allah, or Born Supreme. Many of my friends' names changed overnight: Danny became Supreme; Pumpkin became Messiah; George became K-Star; Evelyn became Queen Aicha; Dana Elain Owens became Queen Latifa.

Even my best friend, Keith, became Rahlik. One honorable trait of the Nation was the principle that your word was your bond. It meant that you couldn't lie under any circumstances, and if your honesty was called into question, all you needed to say was, "My word is bond." It meant you were absolutely telling the truth. "Word is bond" replaced the sayings "I swear on my momma's grave," "I swear on a stack of Bibles," and "I swear on my unborn child."

If there were situations about money, it might go something like this:

"When are you going to pay me back?"

"Next Tuesday."

"Word is bond?"

"Word is bond."

"Here's the money."

One day while I waited for Eddie to bring over more skids, Unique approached the barrels wearing a motherland pendant. I assumed he was waiting for dry towels.

"You righteous?" Unique asked me.

"Nah," I said.

Eddie dropped the skids at my feet. Unique turned to Eddie.

"You righteous?" Unique asked him.

I would've staked my bond—if I had one, that I knew the answer to the question.

"Yep," Eddie said.

Did he really just say he was righteous? I hid my incredulous gaze from Unique, who sauntered away with a dry towel. *If he's righteous, what's his new name?* I wondered. Eddie dumped the slats in one of the barrels and returned to work. Smoke kicked up, sullying the towels, and embers hovered over the barrel like itty-bitty fireworks.

Dirty Caddies and busted Buicks were lined up the block past the used-car lot. The long line delayed our lunch. It also diminished the chance of a cipher, which wouldn't have ended well for Eddie. I thanked Allah.

At lunchtime, I went over the Straight Street bridge for a chicken sandwich from Gene's liquor store. The Kentucky seasoning and RedHot sauce wafted in the air, firing up my taste buds. The fluffy bread stuck to the crumpled aluminum foil. I staved off my impulse to eat in the store and waited till I returned to the car wash. The jokers at the car wash would often ask for a bite of other people's food. I ate outside, where the chance of someone asking for a bite was minimal. If any of the righteous guys wanted a piece, I would claim that there was bacon on it. I munched on my sandwich and tried recalling the names of my coworkers. Avoiding beatdowns was my favorite pastime. Lemme see.

Is it Supreme God cleaning tires or Universe God? No, Universe God is on windows. Supreme God is the one on Armor All duty.

A commotion broke my concentration. Born Supreme and Just God were chasing Eddie. It was only a matter of time before they discovered the truth, leading to the inevitable. They'd caught *righteous* Eddie eating a pork chop sandwich. I should've mentioned that one other thing needed to happen for a beatdown to occur. They had to be able to catch you. I finally figured out what Eddie's righteous name was: Ain't No Way in Hell They Can Catch Me God.

Discarded.

An Odd Year

Mrs. Gardell had taught in the classroom across the hallway from Mrs. Nelson's class. My eyes always ripened whenever Mrs. Gardell would sashay down the hallway in the halo of her Creole beige complexion. And her shape? "Good-gotta-mighty." Mrs. Gardell was 100 percent righteous. So when I discovered she would be my seventh-grade teacher, I actually looked forward to the first day of class.

Lined up in the playground, the first thing I noticed about Mrs. Gardell's voluptuous body was that it was missing. I mean, her head wasn't there either. Someone else's head and body had taken her place. Mrs. Gardell wasn't the only person missing either.

"Anthony Robinson committed suicide," Michael Fields said.

"You lying," I said.

"He hung himself with his fat laces in the bathroom."

"I don't believe you."

Mike punched me in the gut when he told me that. Disbelief spiraled into grief.

"Because he had VD," Mike said.

"What?"

"They said he hung himself because he had VD."

I didn't understand what "VD" meant and didn't ask. Our substitute teacher's introduction cut my bereavement short. Ms. Mitchell's auburn hair blazed above her forehead, making her resemble a circus clown. No one would take her seriously. How long would she be with us? A day? A week? After a month, I stopped guessing. Being new meant Ms. Mitchell was not only white but also green.

After washing every car in Paterson twice, I had saved enough dough to buy my own kicks, and they weren't from a bin at the supermarket. I didn't wear them on the first day of school; only suckers did that. I waited until the second day when it was less sucker-ish.

I pimp-walked down Haledon Avenue rocking my first pair of Pumas, with their blue-on-gray suede joints. I kept a napkin in my pocket for smudges.

"How much they cost?" Nate asked.

"I kicked forty-two ducats for these bad boys."

We had lined up in the schoolyard, preparing to enter the school, when Ms. Mitchell noticed the attention I was receiving.

"What's all the hubbub?" she asked.

"Rodney's new sneakers," Nate said.

Ms. Mitchell looks at them, then nodded.

"Nice. Make sure you don't step on them," she said.

Ms. Mitchell had done her research. She knew rule number one: Never step on a brother's sneakers. She might not end up in a straitjacket after all. Whenever we asked her about Mrs. Gardell's condition, her cheeks would redden. Then she would simply shrug and change the subject. She knew something.

Ms. Mitchell never threatened us with corporal punishment. Deep down, I knew she would've loved to waterboard Wendell Hill and Charles Goodwin. Wendell constantly smacked while chewing his never-ending supply of chocolate Now & Laters. "Please chew with your mouth closed, Mr. Hill," Ms. Mitchell would say.

You think Wendell listened? He smacked even louder. Charles's jokes about her hairdo would've drawn a backhand from Mrs. Nelson or any other Black teacher, but Ms. Mitchell just shook her head and second-guessed her stylist. The thing was, she could've destroyed Charles.

Charles had an extra-long leg. Busting on someone with a malady or an abnormality might've been considered cruel in other places, but not in Paterson. Had she understood the culture, she would've cracked on his mismatched legs. Being white, she would've received extra credit because Black folks "love" to see white people doing Black people shit. Months of heartache could've been avoided from Charles had she said, "I was only pulling your leg. No, wait, someone already beat me to it." But without punishment or any retaliation, Charles ran wild with his joking, keeping everyone tickled pink. Well, the class was tickled. Ms. Mitchell was the only one pink.

Nate and I sat on the stage in the cafe-gym-atorium, listening to Wendell at the end of recess. "If anybody try me, they'll pay a price," he said. Nate made a duck mouth with his hand behind Wendell's back. When I snickered, Wendell's head whipped toward Nate. "Don't make me have to dig in your ass," Wendell said to Nate.

We cracked up. No one took Wendell's bravado seriously. A brawny kid stepped toward us. He inspected each of us as if we had price tags. "Who's the toughest one here?" he asked. In unison, we pointed to Wendell. The dude walked over to Wendell and sized him up. Then struck him in the chest with two quick blows.

"Ooooohhhh," we jeered.

Wendell fell to the floor and curled up like an old caterpillar. The stranger stood over him, like a cocksure man, waiting for Wendell to get up. He looked at us. Who was next? I knew Nate wanted to run. I recognized that look. Wendell writhed in pain, down for the count. The stranger, whose name we discovered was Brandon, left a lasting impression on us and in Wendell's chest.

On the way home, I reminisced about Anthony Robinson. His crazy wide smile and curly 'do. Had Anthony still been living, Wendell might've been spared the agony. I wondered what I would have done if I had been on the receiving end of those two jabs.

Anthony's protection of us died with him in that bathroom. It was rumored he'd been nude when the paramedics found him. The thought of him butt naked with that baby seal swinging was a haunting image. Jokes circulated. *He was hung in more ways than one.* Cruel jokes. Sometimes you can joke about death, but the timing is key. Jaima discovered that bad timing had serious consequences, as you'll soon see.

Discarded.

Frankly Speaking

Frank Mayes rejoined our seventh-grade class following the death of his mom. I could never bring myself to ask how his mom died. My breath grew shallow and tears welled at the thought of losing my mom. I couldn't even finish the thought in my imagination. I was surprised by Frank's spirit, which ran higher than anyone expected. His wisecracks and fish grin put everyone at ease.

Jaima and I sat near each other in class. All the intimacy between us had vanished. It wasn't by my choice; I found out that Alfie had "hit it." A bitterness developed in her that kept other Romeos and me at a distance. Jaima could roll her eyes in a way that stomped our self-esteem. Getting close to her was harder than a seventh-grade boner. Her attitude made dudes call her everything but her government name.

For our industrial arts projects, we had to choose between two designs, a paddle and a fish. A freakin' paddle? To make me build my own paddle was basically sending me to pick my own switch. Guess which one I chose.

Our teacher handed us hacksaws and chunks of wood and left us to our own devices. I locked my block between the jaws of the vice and hacked away, twice a week, until a fishlike figure started taking shape. When the sanding began, so did the jokes.

"What you doing?" someone would ask.

"Buffing the wood. Hacking off. Poking the fish. Shellacking the salmon. Tugging the tuna. Wrestling the eel. Cuddling the catfish. Buffing the blowfish. Filleting the flounder.

Occasionally our teacher looked up from behind his paper, shook his head, and continued reading. He didn't mind us cutting up as long as we didn't cut a finger. And he was a stickler about wearing the protective eyewear. The goofy goggles regularly led to busting.

One day Frank was stroking his salamander on one side of the workshop, while Jaima was poking her fish on the opposite side. Who started snapping first, Frank or Jaima? I don't remember. I do remember who ended it.

"Your ponytail so tight, I can read your mind," Frank said.

The class howled. What happened next was either due to fatigue or perhaps callousness. I thought it was just a lack of creativity. Whatever the reason, Jaima used the default comeback, "Your mother."

All the sanding ceased.

Tiny splinters of wood settled on the Nikes, Pumas, and Hush Puppies. Talking about a person's mother was off-limits unless the joke was vague, but you never, ever talked about a deceased mother. I stopped waxing my dolphin. Even though she could be mean and bitchy, Jaima was still my neighbor and Keith's sister. This was extreme even for her. I leaned over to her.

"Hey, you know that uh…Frank's mom just passed, right?" I told her.

She seemed surprised. "I'll apologize after the class," she said.

The dust settled. I went back to brushing my barracuda, never paying attention to Frank. If I had, I would have seen the tears streaming.

The bell rang. Students stored their chisels and hacksaws. I kicked my sneakers against the wall to remove the remaining sawdust. I walked into the hallway. Frank stood with his back against the wall, eyeing the door. Before I could let him know an apology was on the way, Jaima walked out.

Jaima was either oblivious to or ignored Frank's presence. Frank launched his middleweight frame in the air, throwing a punch that cracked Jaima square in her jaw. She stumbled into the wall, bounced off the plaster, and kept walking as if nothing had happened.

Frank's bouncing movements fizzled, as did his expectation of a fight, a cry, or acknowledgment. We watched Jaima stroll down the hallway without missing a step. Frank looked at me for an answer that I didn't have.

Moments later, in the classroom, I cocked my head to the side, probing Jaima with my eyes as if she were a science project. I couldn't find any bruises or swelling. Encyclopedia Brown had a theory based on Uncle Kenny's perpetual threat as to what had happened. I also had the suspicion that she'd never meant to apologize.

"What you staring at?" Jaima scoffed.

"You know you got punched in the face, right?"

"Who got punched in the face?" Jaima said.

"You."

"Yeah, right. I wish that nigga would."

Uncle Kenny always threatened to knock dice players who left the table early into "the middle of next week." I never believed it was possible, until then. Frank had clearly knocked Jaima into the future. It was the only logical explanation.

Discarded.

Stuck

It was a Monday in October. Only two minutes lay between me and another tardy mark. Too many tardy marks meant a warning notice. I boogied up the stairs, hoping to slide into class before attendance was taken. I eased into class, expecting to hear Ms. Mitchell attempting to gain control of the class, but instead, I was stunned by the presence of Mrs. Gardell.

We called her "Mrs. 1098" because she was a ten dressed to the nines with a figure eight. Out of all my teachers who had laid hands on me, she was the one I would've given permission to. And Mrs. Gardell was socially prominent, not because of her career as a teacher but because of her marriage to a popular pastor.

I would learn a great deal about scandal and shame in the seventh grade. I'd learn a lot about disgrace, Mrs. Gardell's and my own. I'll be a gentleman and start with mine.

A kid in my class named Charles Wright trapped me in an inset doorway. His head and shoulders blocked most of the light coming into the two-by-two-foot cell. Claustrophobia started setting in.

Minutes earlier, before I was trapped, my classmates had been running free in the playground. I tossed my empty bookbag aside and joined the fun. They were playing Garmen, a progressive form of tag where everyone ended up being "it." I juked left and went right, laughing all the while. My shake-and-bake skills broke the ankles of my pursuers, making them look silly. My joy must've maddened Charles Wright. I zigzagged across the playground until I got cornered in the exterior doorway of the industrial arts class.

"You think you funny," Charles said.

His tone killed my smile. I'd thought we were having fun. Everybody was laughing. His fists dangled at his sides; he was about to tag me for real. A crowd of school Twelvers swelled behind him, and the egging started: "Get 'em."

A wide-backed brute, Fella, moved Charles aside. I knew him by reputation only. I couldn't make out his threat due to sensory overload and confusion. I was stuck in a hole, and the darkness was rising. With nowhere to run, I pleaded my case before I suffocated: "Yo, I was just playing. Everybody was playing."

The last thing I saw before the jolt to my right eye, before I fell back into the door, before I covered up, before things went dark, and before the shame, was Fella's smirk.

"Let him go!" someone screamed. Fella wasn't about to let that happen.

My elbow bumped the door behind me. I didn't have enough room to cock my arm—not that I was going to, so I did what I had to do. I panicked.

"If anyone says one more thing, I'm going to fuck him up," Fella said.

Tasha clawed her way through the horde. "Leave my brother alone!" she screamed.

I looked at my sister. "She ain't no kin to me," I said. I was trying to protect her and myself.

The laughter cracked a seam in the blockade, which I slipped through. I high-tailed it home with my unrelated sister in tow. It wasn't over.

When we got home, Mom's cigarette darted in and out of my peripheral vision as she inspected my eye for bruising. She would've had to look deeper than my dark skin to find it. She dumped a few cubes of ice into a towel and pressed it against my eye socket. I grimaced from the bitterness. The freezing water ran down my cheek like frigid tears.

Fella had chumped me in front of everybody with that sucker punch. I could've let it go, but Mom wasn't going to. She told Aunt Doris, who told Uncle Kenny, who told his son Rocky, who told me to get my ass over there.

I hoofed it down to North Fourth street to tell him in person how I'd been jumped. Regrettably, I hadn't spent much time around the Simmonses ever since Mom divorced Howard. How eager would Rocky be to help me? We were still cousins at heart, I hoped.

Rocky leaned on a parked Trans Am, arms folded, highlighting their definition. His creased Lee jeans matched his burgundy do-rag. He noticed my approach then nodded to his boy, who smiled, making me suspicious. Had he already made up his mind? Should I even ask for help?

Rocky's athletic build suited him for the two things he was known for: fighting and flipping. I gave him a pound.

"You heard what happened?" I asked, wanting to know what was being said. Plus, I didn't want to relive the story.

"Nah, not really," Rocky said. He was lying. Nevertheless, I coughed up my account of the altercation. By the time I got to the point where Fella had sucker-punched me, I had realized who was sitting next to Rocky.

Vince's half-shut eye made it appear as if the left half of his face was high and the right half was crazed. More brothers feared him than Rocky. I believed Vince could thrash all three of those punks by his damn self.

"You ready for this, little guy?" Vincent asked. I nodded.

"Don't have us come down there, and you act like a little bitch," Vince said.

"Oh, he won't," Rocky said.

I headed down North Fourth street and saw the corner crowded. I turned around and took the long way home. As an image of Rocky and Vince beating down Fella played in my mind, I grew nervous. Vince's rep for recklessness was well known. He didn't have the normal turn-off switch most sane people have. His switch was dialed way past the level of acceptable violence. People like him were called mad dogs. I doubted Rocky could keep him tame if things went sideways.

The news had spread through school twelve faster than trichomoniasis. Nate and Mike kept asking me if my cousins were coming. "You'll see," I answered.

I didn't know. I'd been asked the question several times throughout the day. Fella was faring better than I had since the gossip about my cousins eliminated the chance of a sneak attack. Only ten minutes remained before the final bell. I started munching on my lip.

Mrs. Gardell's personal issues kept her aloof. She didn't realize what was happening until a student poked her head in our class. "Mrs. Gardell, the principal wants to see Rodney, um…Laney in his office," she said.

Oh shit.

"Oohs" rolled off the puckered lips of my classmates. Evidently, the Kool-Aid grapevine had reached the administration. I stuffed my history and math books into my bookbag since they were the heaviest. I tested the weight. It was capable of inflicting real damage. Mrs. Gardell's subtle expression of concern resonated deeply and gave me the idea of forgiveness. If she could forgive, then anyone could.

Mrs. Presley, the school secretary, spun in her chair to address me or perhaps to see who was behind the commotion. "First time here?" she asked. I nodded. "Make it your last." The commanding woman directed me toward Mr. Booth's office.

Hunched in the corner with clasped hands against his chin sat Fella. He avoided eye contact as best he could. Mr. Booth sat tall behind a desk too big for his office. He extended a long olive-branch arm, pointing toward the empty seat next to Fella, saying, "Have a seat."

I contemplated pulling the seat away from Fella, but I glared at him instead.

"Rodney?" Mr. Booth said.

"Yes," we both said in unison. That sucka's real name was Rodney?

"Laney. What's this I hear about you and your family threatening this Rodney?" Mr. Booth asked me.

"Yesterday, he snuck me for no reason."

"It wasn't me. It was Michael Booth," Fella said.

"It was you," I countered.

Fella pleaded his case to me. I half-listened to his groveling. He blamed Michael Booth—no relation to Mr. Booth—saying he'd reached around him and delivered the blow. *You had me pinned in that doorway*, I thought. After he mentioned it, I recalled seeing Michael Booth peeking over his shoulder with a sinister look. The punch came out of nowhere so fast, I couldn't be sure. All I knew for certain was that he had been standing in front of me when I got walloped, and calling off the mad dog wasn't an option.

"If you're caught fighting on school grounds, you will be suspended immediately, and that will be just the beginning of your problems. Is that understood, Mr. Laney?" the principal told me.

I avoided eye contact with him and swiveled in my seat. I couldn't give a good goddamn since I hadn't planned on fighting. I was leaving that to Vince. Mr. Booth must've had telepathy.

"Whoever fought or *caused* a fight would also get suspended."

Now I gave a little bit of a damn. Mom would skin me alive if I ever got suspended. The principal had put me in a position I couldn't juke my way out of.

I tasted blood from all the lip biting. Standing in front of the doors leading into the playground, I pondered the question: What if it *was* Michael Booth who had sucker-punched me?

The doors opened, and I stepped onto the "stage." To my far left, at the ready, stood a crew with strong resemblances to Fella; their backs were on the wrought iron fence. To my far right, Rocky, Vincent, and their crew, wearing jackets on a day too warm for jackets, huddled on the steps of the chicken coop. Caught in the middle, locked in anticipation, were the school Twelvers. I stepped toward my cousin, headed for redemption.

Vince had come for blood, and it didn't matter whose. It was in his eyes—well, at least one of them.

"What's up?" Rocky asked.

"Um, Fella should be coming out soon," I said.

Vince started shadow boxing, throwing three-punch combinations with insane speed. Before I could ask them not to do what I had asked them to do, a police cruiser pulled up.

"Mr. Booth said I'd get suspended if I caused a fight on school grounds," I told them.

The cruiser's light began swirling, sending a message to the school Twelvers to scatter. Vince was unfazed by the police presence. "They can't stop us from fighting in the street," he said.

The school door clanked opened, grabbing our attention. The two-second walk through the short vestibule and into view was ample time for a prayer. Out walked a substitute teacher. A sigh escaped as I leaned against the chicken coop. Fella was still inside. My prayer had been answered.

The officer blasted his siren, causing the herd to disperse and agitating Vince. "I don't think Mr. Booth is going to let that punk come out," I said. Rocky signaled for his crew to clear out, which they did. All but Vince. He kept eyeing the door.

I parted with Rocky and his crew at the spot at the corner where guys sold drugs. They continued down their path down while I walked uphill, lugging my bag of books.

Mrs. Gardell was carrying an unbearable load. She'd had a nervous breakdown—my first teacher whose nervous breakdown hadn't been caused by her students. It was due to a broken vow. You see, neither the Lord, nor the Church, nor even the congregation could keep Pastor Gardell from cheating on his esteemed wife. According to the rumors, she'd caught her husband home in bed with his lover. "So what?" you might say. "People get caught cheating all the time." Well, he got caught with another man. "OK, it's a little more interesting given the era," you might say, "but still, homosexuality has been around since time immemorial." Yeah, now imagine that Mrs. Gardell not only caught them in the act but had to help them get unstuck.

"What they mean by 'stuck'?" I asked Nate as we sat eating lunch in the cafe-gym-atorium.

Nate sucked down his chocolate milk. "I don't know, but that's what I heard," he said.

Before I learned that dogs could get stuck, I learned that two men could get stuck. They supposedly were taken out on a gurney and then pried apart in the emergency room. Once the Kool-Aid vine got hold of the story, the humiliation for Mrs. Gardell caused a much-needed leave of absence. It was too much for my mind to comprehend. I shirked it off as a heinous rumor.

If Mrs. Gardell's extended absence had been taken with the intention of putting that episode behind her and out of people's minds, she was wrong for two reasons: Charles and Wendell.

"That's why your faggot-ass husband got stuck," Charles said in class one day in response to Mrs. Gardell's cancellation of recess.

I felt such embarrassment for Mrs. Gardell that it was as if Charles had smacked me in the face. I was certain another break-down was looming. After stilling herself, she pointed to the door. "Get the hell out my classroom, Charles." She poised herself with a silent prayer, then gave us worksheets to keep us occupied. I lauded her ability to maintain her composure. It was heroic but didn't feel right. The silence that gripped Mrs. Gardell revealed something crucial. She never denied what was said. It was the lack of denial that made me think the rumor was true. I wondered why she stayed with her husband through it all. Was it faith or forgiveness? I wasn't sure what was needed for someone to leave a marriage, but I thought her situation qualified. It's not like she would've had a problem finding a man.

"I could fill her husband's shoes," Nate joked.

I put my size ten Puma next to his shell-toe Adidas.
"Not like I can."
Discarded.

Donkey Kong

Let's go to Tommy's." One of us inevitably proposed the idea, usually on a dull day. Our friend Tommy Williams had the cure for listlessness. It was the follow-up question that determined our course of action: "You think Mr. Williams is home?"

The Williamses lived at the fringe of Paterson in a working-class neighborhood that bordered the borough of Haledon. A church sat at the top of their block, which made parking impossible on Sundays. A weathered b-ball goal hung above the garage. If our main reason for visiting Tommy didn't happen, playing the Nintendo game Scutter was our second option so long as Ricky, his older brother, wasn't playing.

"Who's going to knock on the door?" I asked.

"I knocked the last time," Kenny declared.

"Let's choose for it," A. T. said.

After three quick thrusts of our fists, I stuck out one finger while they both stuck out two.

"Man, I don't want to walk up there and can't get in," I said.

"You just saying that 'cause you lost," Kenny said.

He was right. Suitors for Bridgette and Baby-Sis, Tommy's sisters, kept their doorbell active, sounding the alarm for their dad. Mr. Williams was a serious, burly man who spoke with a Southern drawl. He made it known by displaying his shotgun that he would inflict harm on anyone out to sin with his girls.

Tommy's harmless nature made him a good fit for our clique. His newly acquired Nintendo had turned his crib into a hotspot. Barrels of laughter awaited us when we could get through the front door.

Mrs. Williams was devoted to the Bible, so we fared better if she answered the door. Mr. Williams's devotion was to his family, and like Donkey Kong, he aimed barrels while we dodged the flames. Facing Mr. Williams produced anxiety for more than one reason.

I surveyed the street ahead, looking for Mr. Williams's car. It sat in their driveway.

"Tommy," Kenny shouted.

I elbowed him in the ribs. "Shut up. You know his father got a shotgun," I said.

"Well, ring the bell then," Kenny said.

"Alright already. Gimme a sec."

The latch for the front gate squealed as I unhooked it. I motioned for Kenny and A. T. to stay out of sight. Chances were better if I was alone. I raised myself up on the balls of my feet to peek through the window, hoping Mr. Williams wasn't on the first floor.

Mr. Williams' negligent boxer briefs didn't do the one job they were made for: to protect onlookers from seeing his dangalang. The first time I'd visited, *it* caught me off guard. I had never really seen a grown man's penis live—a statement I was honored and lucky to make—no thanks to Mr. Blake, the pervert from my old paper route. That day, the head of Mr. Williams's penis snaked out as if to say, "Who ringing the bell?"

I didn't know how to tell Tommy I had been startled by his dad's penis. I was only 50 percent certain Mr. Williams was unaware of what was happening beneath his bulging belly, but I was 100 percent sure I wasn't going to tell him. His dangalang was an effective deterrent.

I mashed the bell and knocked on wood, hoping I wouldn't see any. The Donkey Kong theme music was playing in my mind when Mr. Williams answered the door. *In his mother-freakin' drawers.*

"Is Thomas home?" I asked.

He inspected me as if I were a dog in heat. His slow response made for a long, awkward moment as the head of Medusa swayed in my periphery.

"I know you?"

"Yes, sir. I'm Rodney, Tommy's friend."

Making direct eye contact with men was never my forte, but I made direct eye contact with Mr. Williams. I kept my eyeline above his shoulders.

"Who ya momma?"

"Uh, Valerie," I said.

"Valerie who?" Mr. Williams asked.

"Simmons. Grown-ups call her Kitty."

I heard movement in their kitchen.

"Oh, Kitty. You know Kitty. She works with me at Nabisco," Tommy's mom yelled.

"Oh, Kitty. Yeah, I know Kitty," Mr. Williams said.

The way he said it sounded as if he *really* knew Mom. *Please don't let this man get a woody while saying Mom's name*, I thought.

"Tommy," Mr. Williams called. The yelling caused him to jiggle and increased the chance of a reflex gander by his snake.

"I'll come back later," I said.

"No, just wait here." He called with more force: "Tommy!"

I mean, he had to feel a breeze and the extra leeway. As if things couldn't get worse, he started scratching. *How bad do I want to play this game?* I wondered.

Finally, he adjusted himself. The threat of the turtle head was over. It was only a matter of time before it returned, though. Luckily, Tommy popped out before it did. He waved me upstairs, ignorant of the trauma I had just endured. He demolished me in Donkey Kong. I completely forgot about Kenny and A. T.

Fella started dating Baby-Sis, Tommy's youngest sister. Mr. Williams supposedly warned him to stop coming around. He didn't listen, and Mr. Williams put that shotgun that we were so worried about to use and shot Fella in the chest. As we wondered what would happen to Tommy's father, our Donkey Kong days came to an end. The glimmer in Tommy's eyes had faded a little until he found out that his father wouldn't do any time for killing the other Rodney.

Discarded.

Hot Dogs

Jumping was a game that required a specific skill set. Eric, Alfie, A. T., and I ambled through the neighborhood looking for new heights: a flight of steps, a wall, or a roof. A place where we could climb up and—you guessed it—jump off; a truly cerebral sport. The rules were simple: Anyone who didn't fracture a femur or break a spine won. It was safer than going to Tommy's.

Jumping took heart. It was an exercise in courage. It thrilled the fellas to be daredevils. For me, it was more than daring. For two or three breathless seconds, I was boundless.

One day we chose a ledge atop a roof in someone's backyard—someone who didn't want us there. I gleaned this from the machete that a Puerto Rican man was wielding as he headed straight for us, sidestepping down the narrow ledge. The platform was well over a story high, higher than any of us had anticipated, and the landing was back-breaking concrete.

Eric leaped, then Alfie. The man continued sidestepping, swinging his machete, testing his striking distance. Another yard was all he needed to reach me. It was now or never. The pavement rushed toward me. I tumbled over onto my back, breaking the fall. Then a stinging, as if fire ants were biting into my shins.

A. T. was still on the wall. The man was closing in. I hobbled up, glad I could walk—and, more important, run. "Jump, A. T.," we yelled. A. T. looked at the dude, then the pavement, then back at the dude. "Jump!" we yelled again. The machete slashed at his arm, but it was too late. A. T. landed, tucked, and rolled. Then we jetted up North Fifth street, laughing our asses off.

Nothing works up an appetite quite like a near-death experience. Usually, if Mom wasn't frying chicken or pork chops or baking mac-'n-cheese and cornbread, it was because Freddy had brought home fast food. The smell of sautéed onions in our foyer on this evening told me Freddy had gone to my favorite hot dog spot: Johnny & Hanges. They kept scores of hot dogs sizzling to keep up with the demand for their secret sauce. As I turned the doorknob, I hoped Freddy had remembered to put the sauce on my fries. He surpassed my expectations, bringing home something I would truly relish: a cute honey dip.

Mom and Tasha were waiting to see my reaction, so I played it cool, but the question loomed: *Who is this?*

"This is Marcy, Freddy's niece," Mom said.

"Hi," I said.

"Hello," Marcy said.

Marcy stood. She was five foot eight at least, with curly jet-black hair, the kind you see on the Afro Sheen bottles. With her caramel skin tone, I couldn't be sure if she was all black or half Puerto Rican, but I was certain that she was all deliciousness.

"Oh, he likes her," Mom said, smacking me back to reality. I scoffed at her. *Don't be ridiculous.* I dipped into my room.

"Why don't you take her outside?" Mom called from the kitchen.

"OK. Right after I shower."

"Shower?" Mom asked.

"Where's the iron?" I yelled.

Inside the bathroom, steam fogged the mirror as I showered. When I got out and cleared the condensation, I saw someone I hadn't seen since *that* dreaded day in the fourth grade.

On my way to school twenty-eight, I saw Susan Robinson wearing a dress. You were more likely to see her wearing shoulder pads and a jockstrap than a dress. Timmy was dressed in his Sunday best. Even Alvin was wearing shoes. Dave Beason caught up to me at the corner while I waited on the crossing guard's signal.

"Why everyone so dressed up?" I asked.

"Knucklehead. It's picture day," Dave said.

"For real?"

The photo session took place after recess. I'd worn my everyday clothes and had an expired haircut. The photographer probably knew he wouldn't make money on my pictures.

"Should I say cheese?" I asked.

"It doesn't matter," he replied.

I'd forgotten about the pictures until they arrived. My classmates opened their packages, sneaking peeks and showing their glam shots. Not me.

Once alone in the elevator, I unsheathed the picture from the envelope, shook my head, and stuffed it back in the package. I'd heard the expression: a face only a mother could love. That was about to be put to the test.

Mom opened the packet of photos and shuffled through them as if she were looking for a specific one.

"Jesus. What happened?"

"I forgot it was picture day."

She put them in the back of the photo album. We should've burned them. During a family get-together, Eddie got a hold of the photos, and lo and behold, started in on me: "You big pea-headed bionic-glasses-wearing...."

When he showed the photo to our cousin Tisha, it sparked a visceral gut laugh. Those laughs, those guffaws, spurred my self-doubt and began to frame how I pictured myself.

Now, with Marcy waiting, I cleared the bathroom mirror and began preparing. I dipped into the Sportin' Waves pomade, greased my hair, then brushed my beehive fifty times. I checked my hair for any errant follicles and brushed again. I slipped the blue silk do-rag on and tied it tight. I checked to make sure the circumference of the do-rag was even all around. I thumbed my nose two times. Bruce Lee was ready.

Mom's suggestion to take Marcy outside was well intended, but going out didn't have the impact Mom and I thought it would. Cute Eric, attractive Alfie, and other light-skinned pit vipers were lurking in front of Eric's porch. I kept Marcy on my porch, out of any tournament.

"Runnie," they called.

Sons of bitches wouldn't be sons of bitches if they weren't sons of bitches. And those sons of bitches kept calling me.

"Are those your friends calling you?" Marcy asked.

"Not really" is what I should've said but didn't. We walked toward *my friends*. When we reached them, I stalled the introductions.

"Who is this, Runnie?" Eric asked. A question I'd anticipated but was slow in answering.

"I'm his cousin Marcy," Marcy said.

Cousin. What she mean "cousin"? I did the arithmetic. At most, she was a sister-in-law, which sounded worse. Cousin? That couldn't be right. I double-checked with my dangalang. He said, "No way!"

Good ole dangalang. According to my trusted advisor, we weren't anything but soon-to-be lovers.

Marcy sat on Eric's stoop, stretched her legs, and garnered more attention. There were more dogs in heat around Marcy than at Johnny & Hanges.

Silvia, Nita, and Alphonso, who lived up the hill, walked up, bringing more estrogen and flair to the party. Nita sat on the steps near Eric's Nikes while Silvia rested her parabola-shaped hips against the wall. Alphonso popped his chewing gum, ready to sass somebody. The playing field was momentarily leveled.

Alfie suggested we play Hide and Go Get It, a game where the girls go hide and the fellas go get sexual assault charges. "Nah, nah, homeslice, forget about that," I said. I vetoed his proposal because I knew I would be the only one hiding, while Alfie would be the only one getting it.

"How about a race?" Marcy said.

We all excelled at running except Kenny, who couldn't run to save his life. A. T. joined the challenge, raising eyebrows. Normally, he was too cool to race. Alphonso didn't care to compete, at least not for Marcy, so he set up fifty yards away to be the judge—something he was good at. He spun around, extending his arms to form a lanky finish line. I tightened up my laces.

"On your mark…" Alphonso shouted.

I threw one arm back, Olympian style. Alfie focused on Alphonso.

"Get set…"

I eyed Eric, who was eyeing Marcy, who was eyeing the finish line.

"Go."

Alfie's arms chopped in and out of my periphery. Marcy was gaining. Eric caught up, and the three of us were dogging it. A.

T. dug deep, grimaced, then made his customary Incredible Hulk battle cry: "Grrrrr."

I stretched toward Alphonso's palm, and then it was over. I bent over a few yards past the finish line, gasping in disbelief at who had actually won—it wasn't me. A last-second burst had put the win clearly in the hands of the half-woman, half-gazelle Marcy. The fellas caught their breath while Marcy was ready for another round.

"You must run track," I told her.

"Yep," Marcy said.

"I knew it," Eric said.

"Want a rematch?" she asked him.

"Nah."

Although I'd come in second, my consolation prize came in the form of the news that Marcy was staying the night. Staying the night in my soon-to-be-candlelit bedroom. The only things I needed were candles and my own bedroom.

Later that day, Marcy was chatting and playing with Tasha in the living room. They'd gotten chummy, which was annoying. I had to separate them. I considered striking a match, but Mom was onto my matchbook terrorism. I came up with another plan, but first, I had to use the bathroom.

I took off my do-rag. The waves that roped around my head were so deep, they had seashells. I brushed the sides where the rag was tied to give an even look. There were three reasons I would brush my hair other than for grooming. I stroked my waves when I was vexed, contemplating something or fishing for a compliment. My beehive was the one attribute that drew consistent accolades. It was my secret weapon.

Marcy was popping gum and blowing bubbles like it was her job. I entered the room do-rag-less. She paused her chewing.

"Oh, you got waves for days, huh?" she said.

"These, yeah, I don't really do much. I got Indian in my family," I said.

Marcy got up and stroked her fingers through them.

"Damn, you put a lotta grease, huh?"

"Nah, I just put it in; that's why it's like that."

Marcy wiped her hand on the back of her jeans, then pulled a piece of gum from her back pocket. "You want a piece?" she asked me. She could've offered me rat doo-doo dipped in roach spray, and I would've asked for seconds. She unwrapped it. "Open wide," she said. She placed it on my tongue. Which meant she wanted my babies.

The pipes in our bathroom would rattle when the hot water shut off in the bathroom, and I could hear the noise through the thin wall that separated Tasha's and my closet from the bathroom. That night I sat on the bed, then lay across it, then I sat up again, looking for a cool position while listening for the rattling. I was bracing for the forthcoming glimpse of a freshly showered Marcy.

And then she appeared. Her wet hair was splayed over her shoulders, passing the towel that cocooned her body. She kneeled down to reach into her night bag. *Good-gotta-mighty.* I walked out of the room. I had to.

Sleeping arrangements hadn't been discussed but definitely had been fantasized about. Marcy, I assumed, would sleep with Tasha on the bottom bunk, while I would sleep on the top in my pup tent.

"Do you mind if Marcy sleeps in your bed?" Mom asked. *Hell no*, I thought. Way to go, Mom. "Good, then you can sleep on the sofa," she said. *Oh, you meant...?*

"What's your name?" Aunt Mildred asked Marcy.

"Marcy."

Freddy had taken us over to Uncle Butch and Aunt Mildred's home. Aunt Mildred stroked Marcy's hair in her foyer, saying, "So pretty." The compliment reddened Marcy's cheeks. I delighted in her modesty. Uncle Butch led Freddie to the man's terrain in the backyard.

"Eddie!" Aunt Mildred shouted upstairs before she and Mom went into the kitchen.

"This is a nice neighborhood," Marcy said.

"It is," I replied.

"I want a house like this one day," Marcy said.

Eddie hopped down the flight of carpeted stairs, landing with a thud.

"Who is this?" Eddie asked.

"Freddy's niece," I said.

"Freddy's niece got a name?"

"Marcy," Marcy said.

Eddie stuck out his hand, saying, "I'm Eddie."

Marcy shook his hand for way too long.

"Want to see something cool?" Eddie asked.

Marcy nodded, following Eddie as I followed her. Our host guided us to the corner of the living room, where an illuminated fish tank housed two piranhas. "They still haven't eaten yet," Eddie said. A goldfish poked its fat lips out of his fish cave house in the corner. He knew piranhas were lurking in those waters. Two maneaters bided their time.

"The big one usually will eat first. The smaller one only eats when there's more than one," Eddie said. He tapped the tank, instigating a brawl. The piranhas livened up. Marcy covered her eyes while we waited for the frenzy. The big-eyed goldfish swam out of the cave. I guessed he figured you can't run in a fishbowl. To Eddie's confusion, though, the killers didn't attack. It's hard to perform when everybody's watching.

"There is definitely something fishy going on here," I said.

Marcy chuckled. Eddie shrugged, then walked over to his basement door and waved for us to follow. Eddie's home never seemed larger. Downstairs, the pool table covered the majority of the lair. Uncle Butch's favorite recliner sat at one end of the table while the washer and dryer stood in the corner. Eddie chalked a stick while I started collecting balls from the pockets. The chances of my beating him were slim since he'd taught me how to play.

Eddie asked Marcy if she wanted to play, and of course, she did, so he gave her a stick. Eddie leaned against her as he went over the rules of the game. I pulled out my hairbrush. He showed her how to aim and stroke the cue while I stroked my beehive in all directions. Marcy blew bubbles with her gum while Eddie racked up. I dropped into the La-Z-Boy like an oddball in the side pocket.

On the ride home later that day, Luther Vandross inspired me once again.

When we got home, Freddy, Mom, and Tasha walked into our apartment. Before Marcy could go inside, I poked her in her side, motioning for her to stay on the porch. When the door shut, she stood with me. She expected me to say something, but poking her was all that I had been planning. She took her gum out of her mouth.

"It's my last piece. Want a bite?" she asked.

Due to my keen ability to detect overtures, I said: "I can get you some more."

Marcy curled the gum around her finger that was swirling right below her dimple, then she plucked it into the air.

"Let's walk to the store. I'll get you some more," I said. We descended the staircase shoulder to shoulder. Her hand brushed mine as my heart raced toward the finish line. I turned Marcy toward me and pressed my lips to hers. Her tongue, a welcome surprise, made me victorious. I floated in the winner's circle breathless and boundless. I had to pry myself away from her. She felt too damn good. I wanted to run up the block and let the fellas know: *I kissed Marcy.*

It was time to say something. I knew that because Marcy said, "Say something." I knew whatever I said would've been stupid: "Your kiss makes me want to do jumping jacks. Do you still want gum? My penis is hard enough to chip a diamond."

A call from the porch saved me. "Marcy!" Tasha yelled.

We released our hold and separated. "Go see what she wants. I'll run to the store," I said. Marcy answered the call, and I adjusted my drawers.

Cousins we were not. I sailed up Haledon Avenue on my way back without looking up at Morny and Raquel's perch. I was too busy planning the next kiss. My options for locations were the overgrown bushes behind the apartments or our basement with the romantic scent of mildew.

At our door, I stuffed the candies into my pockets. If Mom saw the bag of candy, it would arouse suspicion. She knew I didn't eat much candy. The empty living room jolted me. I heard Mom in the kitchen on my way to the bedroom. It was empty.

"Where did Marcy go?" I asked.

"Freddy took Marcy back home," Mom replied.

What?

I hadn't even gotten her number. I shut the door to my room and lay on my black hole of a bed. I emptied the contents of my pocket, then popped Boston Baked Beans candies as if they were antidepressants. *Surely Freddy will bring her back one day*, I thought.

But that would've required Mom and Freddy to stay together, which they didn't.

I worked up the nerve to ask Mom what happened with Freddy for my own selfish reasons. "Freddy doesn't want anything. And I want a house," Mom said. At that moment, I thought, *A woman would never leave me for not owning my own home.*

Discarded.

Medication

One Saturday morning during the summer, Kenny pushed me off my bike, and when I fell, I heard a loud pop in my left leg. I tried to stand but toppled. I leaned on A. T.'s shoulder all the way home. When Mom rolled up my pant leg, we saw that my knee had swollen to the size of a grapefruit. The sight of it caused more agony than the actual injury. Mom went to get a painkiller.

"Take these pills," she said.

"I'm fine," I said.

"Take 'em."

Mom's Laney scowl surfaced. My unwillingness to take the white pills confused Mom. My reasoning stemmed from someone else's injury.

After Mom and Freddy broke up, so did Aunt Mildred and Uncle Butch. Aunt Mildred moved into a one-bedroom unit in an apartment complex in Hackensack. One day my Mom dropped me off at the curb, and I followed the stairs leading up to a square patio. I hadn't seen Eddie in weeks and was eager to hear about his latest conquests. Hackensack girls were known for being hop-in-the-sack chicks.

I checked the address number on my sheet against the numbers on the green doors until I found the one that matched. I rang the bell, and a fat-head dude opened the door.

"Oh, sorry, I got the wrong address," I said.

"It's me," Eddie said.

Eddie's head had doubled in size. My open mouth revealed my bemusement.

"It's the medication. I had an allergic reaction," Eddie said.

I shouldn't have been so surprised that day. Whenever Eddie visited me in Paterson, I would count the seconds before he asked, "Want to shoot hoops?" Often we would go to Brooks Sloate, the least violent project in Paterson, where we could get a run on the courts without ending up in one.

On one of Eddie's visits, we hiked up North Seventh to West Broadway, talking smack the whole way. Eddie had taught me how to shoot both pool and hoops, so I marked my progress by how well I played against him. After we got there and started a game with the guys, Eddie hit a jump shot from the top of the key. He had the hot hand, and no one could guard the southpaw that day. We were on the same team and needed only one more bucket for the win. Eddie took the inbound pass. I ran up court looking for the long pass. Eddie dribbled a few yards before stopping at center court. He grew alarmed, then let the b-ball drop. It rolled toward the sideline. He sprinted straight toward me.

"We gotta go. We gotta go," Eddie said.

"What's wrong?"

He ran past me headed toward home, which was at least a mile away. I charged after him. By the time I caught up to him, all he could do was point at his wide-open mouth.

"Ah kant shuh muh maa," he said.

"What?" I said.

"Ah kant shuh muh maa."

We were playing high-speed charades. I figured out that he couldn't shut his mouth, but there was no prize. Eddie did what he always did in a crisis: started laughing. We were ass and elbows running home, leaving a trail of his drool in our wake.

Now, back at home with my grapefruit-size knee, I saw two white globular masses of something with unknown consequences in Mom's palm.

"You sure you don't want to take these?" she asked.

"I'm sure."

I'd rather have a swollen knee than a fat-ass head.

Discarded.

Mr. Miller

The elderly man had an S Curl, a greasy hair texturizer designed to make his appearance more youthful. It did not. The thick mat of hair on his head connected to his grizzly sideburns that ran into a goatee. Two shaggy eyebrows completed his bushy look. A pair of gold herringbone necklaces choked his Adam's apple. Sharp creases ran down the middle of his pants straight into his shiny boots. Mr. Miller was sitting cross-legged in our living room.

Mr. Miller's popularity came from the restaurant he'd once owned: Miller's Diner. The ex-restaurateur shook my hand with a callused palm and a surprisingly solid grip for an old-timer.

"You need to firm up that grip, young man. Let's try it again," Mr. Miller said. He kept eye contact while nodding in approval over my stronger grip. Giving his fuzzy face the once-over, I wondered if he was genuinely interested in me or if it was simply a show to impress Mom.

Mr. Miller, aka Bob, lasted with Mom past the expiration date I gave him. He even started coming around out of his moving company's uniform, a risky move. He wore a jean motorcycle gang jacket that read "Iron Horseman" across the back. He spoke of having ridden with bikers, but he no longer owned a bike. The only things that remained of his restaurant and bike-riding days were the stories he told in his deep, scraggly voice. I leaned into his stories, particularly if a shot of "Knotty Head," or gin, preceded the telling. If the motorcycle club wasn't the theme, then Betsy, his truck, was.

"You gotta know how to make tight turns when ya drive a straight bed. It ain't as easy as driving an eighteen-wheeler," he would say.

Often I wanted to say, "How hard can it be? It's a truck," but I knew he didn't have Freddy's sense of humor. He drove for the Vernay franchise of North American Van Lines, a moving company whose warehouse was at the end of Governor Street. According to him, he was the head honcho of his team, handling the paperwork, money, and hiring of extra hands. The last part of his responsibilities made me glad I didn't mock him.

One day Mom opened the door to my room and stood there. I snapped to attention and started straightening up, waiting for the "Clean up this room" lecture. Her sunny gaze said it wasn't about the mess. Something else was on her mind.

"Bob wants to know if you'd be interested in working with him," she told me.

"On the moving truck?"

"Where else?" I understood her hesitation now.

"Think about it," Mom said.

"OK," I said.

"OK as in you'll think about it, or OK as in you'll do it?" she asked.

"I'll do it."

"You sure?"

"Yeah, I'm sure."

Mom closed the door with a nod of approval. I'd lied. I wasn't sure. The cheeriness had left her when I hesitated, and I didn't like being the cause of that.

I marveled at Mr. Miller's stories about the "byways and highways" and the "purposes and the accidents." I wanted my own road stories to tell, but I also learned that wanting something badly was the quickest way to a wreck. I remembered Uncle Kenny's promise to take me to work with him on his sanitation truck, and how that broken promise left me feeling like garbage. I reined in my hopes and lay on the bed, refusing to be let down again.

Mom opened the door again.

"Bob said he'll be picking you up around six a.m. Saturday morning. Y'all going to Virginia." *Virginia—three states away.*

The early morning's radiance that Saturday reflected in Mom's smile as she waved. I chomped on the last bite of my egg-and-bacon sandwich, headed toward the straight truck. I followed behind the dangling keys and freshly pressed uniform of Mr. Miller. The passenger cab door swung open. A frail man trembled down onto the pavement, followed by another man who hopped out to make room for me. They wore light blue North American shirts and dark blue khakis. The frail man stuck out his hand.

"Joe Blue," he said.

I made sure to give him a firm grip. "Rodney," I said.

The agile man stuck out his hand. "Jimbo," he said.

His handshake was weak. He obviously hadn't received the lecture from Mr. Miller. I pulled myself into the cab and straddled the stick shift to make room for Joe and Jimbo. The engine growled when Mr. Miller shifted the truck into gear, jerking us into traffic and making Jimbo's and my shoulders bump. Every time the gear shifted, our knees knocked. I looked out of the corner of my eye at Jimbo for traces of irritation, but he was breezy. Nope, it didn't bother Jimbo one bit.

I thought it funny that a guy with bloodshot eyes and tan teeth would be named Joe Blue. And those weren't his most colorful attributes. The most colorful was his raspy voice that was stained with alcohol. I figured he was smart since Mr. Miller asked his opinion about routes. And Jimbo, let's just say he was definitely the brawn of the trio. Jimbo and Joe were Mr. Miller's number one and number two, and over the next few weeks, I intended to become his number three.

When we got to the place where we'd be working, Jimbo hopped out of the cab to guide Mr. Miller into his parking space. I observed Mr. Miller crank the wheel and shift gears, all while riveted to his rearview mirror. After Jimbo gave the thumbs-up, Mr. Miller pulled a red lever, releasing a hiss of air. The wonderment in my face led him to offer an explanation.

"That's the air brake. See, you got three brakes—one right here."

He stepped on a large pedal on the floor, then grabbed another handle.

"One right here. I popped this one here with the red button. You see, you need a lot of compressed air to stop Betsy from rolling. Then there's a release valve under her skirt that makes the brakes stick."

"What makes that sound?" I asked.

"That's the air escaping the brake valve."

"Interesting."

Mr. Miller grabbed his clipboard, twisted his cigarette out in the ashtray, then double-checked his shirt pocket for his gold pen. It was time to work.

Mr. Miller, a poised man, rarely let his S curled hair down. We were working for a single fortysomething white woman who was relocating to Virginia. She was moving into a two-story condo in a spread-out condominium complex. The manicured grounds posed the first issue since they prevented us from backing the truck up to the doorway. Being able to unload there would've kept the 7,000-pound job quick and easy, but since each piece of furniture had to be carried from the curb up a long sidewalk to the house fifty yards away, it took the time of an 18,000-pound job. I didn't mind as much as the others since I was getting paid by the hour.

Joe Blue wobbled over to the back of the truck. Jimbo grabbed his hand, pulling him up. Then Jimbo hopped down, and Joe pushed the furniture to the edge. Jimbo and I saddled up and hauled each piece over half a football field to the front door's step, without stopping.

The Virginian heat worked overtime on us. Sweat drizzled from my forehead onto the boxes filled with old books I was certain the lady was never going to read. My back and shoulders began to throb.

Intent on keeping her new pad spotless, the client tracked us with her spray bottle. *Squish, squish, squish* went the spray trigger. She pulled the trigger on dust mites, lint balls, or any possibility of dirt. When Mr. Miller and I trudged up with the sofa, an agonizing trip, we found the door closed. He huffed and sighed, engaging his personal air brakes. He balanced the sofa on his knee to free up one hand to slide the door open.

"You gotta keep the door open, ma'am, so we can do our jobs," he told the lady. She mumbled something about the cost of central air and went about squishing.

Later on, the door was locked again, sparking a cigarette break. The S Curl's activator, the chemical designed to make the curl appear wet, dripped down Mr. Miller's neck into his shirt as his

S-Curl glistened in the sun. "We should drop the furniture on her steps and tell her to kiss our ass," Joe Blue said.

Mr. Miller took a long pull on his cig, and I wondered if that was really an option. "Break over," he said.

I walked adjacent to Mr. Miller as we headed into the apartment through the back entrance. The cigarette had apparently topped off his patience. He was advising me on how to handle clients that ruffle feathers when his face whipped to the right as if a chiropractor had snapped his neck. The clonk stunned me as well. Then I realized what had happened.

The sliding glass doors we assumed were open *were not*. Mr. Miller's bushy face had smashed into the door. S-Curl juice slopped against the pane glass, leaving a greasy outline of an angry black man.

"I told you to keep the damn door open," Mr. Miller yelled. He started a wild rant. I listened, but not really. I was focused on stifling my laughter. A chuckle slipped out of my throat. Mr. Miller's eyes and anger locked on me. *This shit ain't funny*, he was clearly conveying. As we walked back to the truck, I felt him watching me, waiting for me to slip. I didn't want to lose the gig, but the image of his face kept replaying in my mind—that second of terror on his face before he realized what had happened. He'd probably thought he had a heart attack. I bit hard on my lip, fighting to compress the air bubbling in my chest. My lips quivered. I turned and made a break to the apartment, found a half bath downstairs, released the valves, and started rolling. When I closed the door behind me, all I heard was *squish, squish, squish*.

Then it was lunchtime. With the CB handle "Soul Food," it was no surprise that Mr. Miller knew all the best truck stops. Joe Blue didn't order food; he ordered cuisine: clams on the half shell with white sauce. Jimbo ordered fried chicken, then showered it in Louisiana Red Hot sauce. Our family never dined out, so I copied what Mr. Miller ordered. I saw him spread his napkin over his lap and did the same. When my plate landed in front of me, I held off for a second and learned truckers didn't pray; they dug in.

On the drive back to New Jersey that night, the drone of the diesel engine knocked out Joe and Jimbo. Mr. Miller cracked his window and lit a cigarette. The night air whistled and breezed along the nape of my neck, stirring me out of sedation. He pointed at the shoulder of the road.

"If you find yourself on a dark road, keep your eyes on the white lines. As long as you know where those lines are, you'll stay on the road," Mr. Miller said.

My eyes followed those lines along the embankment until they blurred. I fell asleep knowing Mr. Miller would keep me on the right side.

A tug at my shoulder jolted me back to consciousness.

"Huh?" I said.

"We're here," Mr. Miller said.

I peeled my cheek off Mr. Miller's shoulder, wondering how long it had been resting there and hoping he didn't mind.

"Thanks, Mr. Miller," I said.

"You can call me Bob, young man," Mr. Miller said.

"Thanks, Bob."

Discarded.

Man Up

The front door slammed at eleven something on a Friday night. Mom was fired up. I widened the crack of my bedroom door, contemplating any wrongdoing I might have done, but nothing came to mind. Mom's shadow stretched out from the bathroom and ran into her bedroom door. Every time it moved, something slammed against the sink or medicine cabinet. She was preparing for battle.

I had to peek. I stood in Mom's shadow as she tucked her hair underneath a cap, then smeared a heap of Vaseline over her face. She felt my presence but ignored it. Only after rolling up her sleeves did she look at me.

"You coming?" Mom said. I nodded. "Come on then."

Trying to stop her never crossed my mind, but it would've if I had known who she was going after. She marched down the steps. I trotted, walked, and trotted again to keep pace.

"I'm going to whoop Mary's ass," Mom declared.

Mary? As in Rocky's girlfriend, Mary? As in Rocky's baby momma Mary? Mary, the one with the two brothers? That Mary?

I'd heard the story before, usually when Mom was nursing a migraine or after a night of puking. The wretched women in the motorcycle club she went to with Bob underestimated her because they thought she was drunk, due to her sleepy eyes, not realizing that Mom's sleepy appearance was due to her having been born without muscles in her upper eyelids. Their presumption about her eyes caused their own to become blackened—by Mom. They would leave the club saying, "Damn, that drunk-ass woman could fight."

Mary lived two houses down from our complex on the first floor of a two-family house, with only a small porch and no front yard. Going to her house violated the primary rules. Never go to someone's home to fight; always find neutral ground. Never drink before a fight, which Mom had clearly been doing. And the most important rule—which I made up while walking behind her—was never go to a house where a lot of men live who could possibly thrash your son. It became obvious these rules never made it to South Carolina when Mom started banging on Mary's door.

I assumed Mary was in her house picking up a bat, a chain, and a wrench and weighing her options on which would draw the most blood. Mom raised herself up to her tippy toes to peek into the hallway. I focused on the doorknob. We were seconds away from being butchered to death. She knuckled the door again. I knew they'd damn sure heard her that time. This was it.

"What did she do?" I asked.

"She was talking shit on me."

She was talking shit on you? Cursing wasn't Mom's forte, but I got the point. She hammered again, then backed away without backing down. Out of all the people who lived in that house, no one was home.

Mary was related to Bob. Through Mom's grunts and mumbles, I discovered that he was somehow mixed up in the drama. And although Mom didn't put her foot in Mary's ass, Bob got the boot.

"You won't be going on any more trips with Bob," Mom said.

It was a gut punch I hadn't seen coming.

Discarded.

Eastern Christian

Eastern Christian, a private Christian school in Haledon, had a basketball court with a high vacancy rate and a water fountain that shot cold water high enough to hit a three-pointer. It became our eighth-grade afterschool hangout because it was the nearest basketball court to our apartments, even though it was off-limits, reserved for Haledon residents only. A policy designed to keep "Us" Patersonians away.

Supreme, Danny's new righteous name, had stuck gum on the sprout, causing the stream to blast Eric in the face. Eric wiped the water out of his nostril while Supreme and I pointed at him, slapping our thighs. Eric paid little attention to our chuckles; something above the water fountain had his attention. A plan began sprouting.

After a few games of Scutter, popularly known as Twenty-one, we ventured over to the Double Dragon restaurant for iced tea and chicken wings. I squirted a copious amount of duck sauce on my egg roll while listening to Supreme and Eric scheme. They were still yapping about it when we left as we walked up North Eighth street and down Haledon Avenue. I didn't think we would actually go through with it, but then it was nightfall, and we were heading back to the school.

What could we possibly gain from breaking into a school? How much time in juvie would we get if we got caught? What would the police do to three young black boys caught stealing? These are the questions I should've asked before hopping up on the fountain and slipping through the window.

We stood in the dim hallway looking at each other, confused about what to do next. That's as far as the plan went. We improvised, meaning we zigzagged to each classroom, looking for anything worth taking. A telephone with a built-in recorder caught my attention. I turned to get an opinion, but Eric and Supreme had skated. Sticking together wasn't part of the plan, I guessed. Their plundering echoed in the hallways. Cat burglars, we were not. I followed the commotion until my intuition stopped me. *Get out now*, it demanded.

I scurried through the building, looking for Supreme. I found him in a room that resembled our home economics classroom.

"Let's get out of here," I said.

Back at our entry point, I poked my head out the window, hoping it wouldn't get blown off by Prospect Park's finest. The coast was clear. I let Supreme hop out first since he was carrying two sewing machine cases. The wide-open playground made us too visible, so we stayed close to the building until we reached a staircase that stretched from the building's north side down to North Seventh street. The sewing machine scraped the walls as Supreme rambled down the steps and blindly darted out onto the sidewalk.

"Don't move!" someone yelled.

A cop stood outside his cruiser a few yards away with his gun drawn. He had ordered Supreme to stop, which is exactly what he didn't do. Uncertain if the cop saw me, I flattened myself against the wall. Supreme teeter-tottered downhill.

"Stop," the policeman ordered.

Certain that gunfire would be next, I shot back up the stairway until I reached the landing. If the police discovered the open window by the fountain, I was done. I glanced back to see if the cop was approaching from my rear; no gunshots yet. That was good. I scoped the playground—nothing but darkness.

Another siren signaled that more cops were coming. I cut across the open playground, trying to look innocent while carrying a stolen phone. *If I make it to Double Dragon, I'll order an egg roll and rib tips to blend in*, I thought.

I crossed North Eighth Street. A police cruiser passed the corner headed toward North Seventh Street. I bailed on the egg roll and hightailed it up North Eighth. I ran through the funeral home parking lot and dipped into the bushes of Mr. Willie's backyard, panting. I was home free but couldn't breathe easy knowing that Supreme might be in custody or worse.

I hid the phone in my shirt and jogged home. A. T. and Kenny were being held captive on the stoop by the story Eric was already telling.

"You see Su?" I asked Eric.

"Nah."

"We gotta go back," I said.

"You must be crazy," Eric said.

"The cops showed up, and...and all I heard was 'Don't move.'"

Kenny stood, while A. T. remained on the stoop.

"You better hide that phone first," A. T. said.

Before I could figure out what to do with the loot, someone approached me from behind, jogging down the parking lot. I turned to see his gold grin.

"You looked like a damn penguin running with those big-ass machines," I said.

"Do you still get to make a phone call if you get caught stealing a phone?" Supreme said.

"If those cops would've caught yo ass, you coulda made your own stitches," I answered.

Discarded.

Tomas

Going into my house was never a casual affair for several reasons. The main reason was that I never knew if I would be allowed to leave. My freedom was dependent on Mom's discretion and mood. Only after I had severe dehydration did I risk going in the house after 5 p.m. What awaited on the other side of the door was always a mystery.

I entered our living room to discover a bug-eyed, dark-skinned, ham-hock-eating player sitting behind a whisky glass. Tomas made Bob look like Billy Dee Williams. Tasha and I understood that Mom didn't care about looks, but didn't she realize we also had to look at him? Talking to Tomas was arduous because he was a mumbler, and his speech slurred whenever he drank—which was every time I saw him. Tomas wore fashionable button-up shirts and slacks but no uniform. Only severe hunger pains could make me go home to stomach Tomas's mumbling. On this night, they overrode my reluctance to squint and nod and fake understanding his gibberish.

It was after 5 p.m. when I twisted the doorknob to find Tomas, who was utterly unaware of my entrance—either because of his stupor or because of the Ginsu knife pointed at his gut. I guessed the latter.

"Please, baby, please!" Tomas begged.

"Get out," Mom said.

Tomas held up his arms in the "Don't shoot" position.

"I'm not going to tell you again," Mom warned.

Tomas's toughest challenge at that point was standing erect, or maybe it was avoiding the tip of that blade. It was a toss-up.

"Please, baby, I didn't mean no harm," he said.

"Get out."

Oddly enough, I didn't feel any alarm. Then again, I wasn't about to get shanked. My ease came from Mom's matter-of-fact tone. But as drunkards do, regardless of a potentially life-ending threat, Tomas took a step forward. Mom didn't step back.

"I'm going to tell you one last time. Get out of my house," Mom said.

Mesmerized by Mom's dreamy eyes, Tomas took another step. And there is where he met the knife. Luckily for him, it was a superficial acquaintance. Blood trickled down his arm. Feeling the sting, I grimaced. Tomas, too drunk to feel anything, lurched forward. Mom gave him a last warning slice. She was about to start poking this fool. I knew it, Mom knew it, and thank God Tomas realized it. He backed out the door I was holding open and staggered into oblivion.

After washing off Tomas's blood from her knife, Mom plunked down on the couch and unrolled her sleeves. I sat at her feet, waiting to see what we were going to watch on TV.

A week or so later at 5 p.m., I stood on the porch with cotton mouth; I was approaching renal failure. I sighed and turned the doorknob.

"Hey there, young man," I heard.

Bob stood to greet me. I gave him a sturdy handshake and stayed inside the rest of the night.

Discarded.

Broken Codes

K-Star, a recent convert to "righteousness" who started hanging in "the Dead End," knelt in the bushes behind the funeral home parking lot, aiming, with his finger on the trigger. I knelt next to him, second-guessing my decision to give him my BB gun. K-Star swayed his aim, tracking his six-foot-four mark: a guy named Messiah. *Bang!* Dead on target. K-Star shot Messiah simply because he thought he could get away with it.

Mr. Willie's dog barked, giving our position away. We flew out of the bushes like scared crows. We ran to "the dead end," where K-Star chucked the BB gun down the steps behind A. T.'s stoop. Then we pretended to have been sitting there all along as if nothing had happened, as if K-Star hadn't just shot Messiah right between his eyes with a pellet. I forced my diaphragm to become steady and tried to breathe normally, so I wouldn't draw suspicion.

Mike, Messiah's pipsqueak cousin, rolled down the hill on his bike. "They down here," he called.

Messiah galloped down the hill straight toward us. "Who shot me?" he said. His interrogation drew dumb looks from K-Star and me. *How would we know?* Messiah's eyes shifted between us, searching for guilt.

A *click-click* sound came from Mike's bike as he peddled in reverse. He was a buzzard circling. Behind our backs was a five-foot drop into A. T.'s basement. A shove from Messiah would plunge us onto the jagged steps below. I slid my hands underneath my legs to hide my grip on the stoop. A knot bulged in K-Star's throat as Messiah moved closer. Blood was trickling from the bridge of his nose.

"Who shot me?"

"Not me," K-Star said.

"K-Star" wasn't his government name; K-Star was righteous. Meaning he was supposed to live up to the higher standards set by the Five Percenters. But that lie was 100 percent ordinary. I wanted to say, "Negro, you know damn well who shot him."

"I saw who did it. He was wearing a white shirt," Mike shouted. He'd broken the code by committing an act done only by the scummiest backstabber: He was snitching, and I couldn't have been happier because I wasn't wearing a white shirt. I couldn't say the same for K-Star, whose bright white shirt was soaking with sweat.

"I didn't do it," K-Star said.

Messiah grunted. His breathing became erratic and choppy, and his anger bled through his eyes. His long arms were cocked with hard-hitting fists. One of us was about to get sledgehammered.

"I know it's your gun, Rodney," Messiah said.

I knew I shouldn't have taken that damn BB gun.

I had gotten it on my last job with Bob, which turned out to be a nice payday. It didn't have anything to do with the payload. While I was fishing around in the client's attic for a box to put on the hand truck, a metallic rod pierced the dimness. Standing tall in a dusty corner was the barrel of a shotgun. The caked-on dust made it appear old, but after some rubbing, it shone like new. I took aim at my imagination, seeing how terrified anyone on the opposite end of that gun would be. I laughed. In the corner, another gem awaited. I picked up a switchblade with a leather thong hanging from the handle. I flicked my wrist to see the long, sharp blade. Etched in the handle in gold lettering was "007." James Bond was the ultimate ladies' man. Mom adored herself some Sean Connery.

"That's a good-looking white man," she would say.

The fellas would get a kick out of these weapons, I figured. I put them back in their place, then loaded my hand truck. I put the knife and gun into a cloth tarp and wrapped it in a rubber band. I didn't pack it until the truck was nearly full. Then I stashed it in a crevice over the wheel well, where I could retrieve it easily. *Would they even be missed?* I wondered.

Now, sitting on A. T.'s stoop, I was about to pay for it.

"It's your gun, Rodney," Messiah said.

"It wasn't me."

"Then who was it?" Messiah asked. I kept quiet.

"It's your gun," Messiah said again. He inched toward me.

"Whoever did it was wearing a white shirt," Mike repeated.

I had the inclination to scream, "Listen to your cousin! Which one of us is wearing a white shirt?" but I suppressed it. Finally, it clicked in Messiah's mind. He wound up, ready to bust K-Star's ass. Relief swept over me. *Yeah, bust* his *ass.*

"Word is bond. I didn't do it," K-Star said.

My head snapped toward him in disbelief. Mike slid his bike to a halt. Had he just stated, "Word is bond"? He'd broken his righteous oath. Unfortunately, only I knew it. K-Star couldn't look at me after that, but it didn't matter since Messiah had his eyes aimed at me.

"It's your gun, Rodney," Messiah said.

K-Star had broken his bond. Mike had snitched. Why shouldn't I? I sighed, shook my head, and stood up. "Let's take it up the hill," I requested.

Fights never took place in front of the apartment building, an unspoken rule. We walked a few yards uphill to Carbon Street. In the middle of the street, traces of blood trickled from the top of Messiah's nose bridge. Messiah threw up his fists, and I put up my guard. Whenever Messiah boxed, he threw long-armed, windmill haymakers that crashed through all defenses. Because of the length of his arms, even if his blows missed your head, they still hammered your back.

I held my ground, waiting to duck.

"I can't fight you," Messiah said. He dropped his dukes, turned, and walked home. His pipsqueak cousin cycled behind him. Messiah had spared the Rod.

That gun brought me more trouble than it was worth, but it was nothing compared to the severity of the 007.

Discarded.

The Slicing

The night of the move where I'd picked up my new weapons, I snuck out of the house after I was certain Bob was in for the night. He'd parked the truck on North Seventh Street, a block away from the house. I had left the back of the truck unlocked so I could retrieve the BB gun and the knife. I got them from their hiding place, clicked the padlock shut, gave a tug to make sure it was secure, then took my trophies home.

The long blade of the 007 clicked into place with a quick snap of my wrist. I couldn't imagine actually stabbing someone. The Pablos, Pacos, and Pedros were known to carry knives, but real men handled business with their hands. I taped the switchblade to the side of my bed that faced the wall. I slept comfortably with my new security blanket.

Days after the Messiah event, I bopped up to A. T. and Kenny, who were slumped forward on the stoop in front of Eric's apartment. Their flat expressions meant they were primed for the big reveal. I hid both weapons until I got close enough to put the muzzle on A. T.'s shoulder.

"Don't move," I said.

"Yooo, let me see that," A. T. said.

"I know that ain't real," Kenny said.

I handed the gun to A. T., then snapped the switchblade open and waved the two guys apart to make room for me. After they slid to the side, I took my place between them with the blade of the knife jutting straight up from my lap.

"Is that a double-oh-seven?" Kenny asked.

"Yep."

"Where did you get it?" Kenny continued.

"Don't worry about that," I said.

A. T. took aim at the garbage shed.

"Don't shoot it," I ordered.

"Let me see that thing," Kenny said.

I folded the steel shank and passed it to him. "Feel the weight on that bad boy," I said.

Kenny nodded in agreement. "You could really do damage with this," he said.

"A. T., let Kenny check out the gun," I said.

They exchanged my new tools while I sat erect, enjoying their adoration. A. T. handed back the 007. Eric came out of his house, then hopped off his porch.

"Let me see that," Eric said.

I gripped the 007 so the blade pointed upright. Perhaps there wasn't enough respect in Eric's tone, or maybe it was because it sounded more like a demand than a request, but whatever the reason, I wasn't in the mood to let Eric see my dagger. I shook my head no, slowly.

"Let me see the knife?" Eric said.

"No."

"Come on, I just want to hold it."

"I said no."

Eric then grabbed the *blade* of the knife. Who in their right mind grabs the blade of a knife? Eric, that's who.

"Let me see it."

"You better let go of the knife, Eric," I warned him.

He wouldn't let go. His cockiness challenged my manhood. I yanked it from his grasp, slicing his finger. He yelped in agony and disbelief. Normally he would've taken a swing at me, but the knife with his blood on it remained pointed at him, so he ran into his house. Everyone knew it wasn't over.

His mom's yelling promised more drama. If his mom was trying to calm him, she failed. The door swung open. Eric leaped off the porch, charging toward me. He was brandishing what appeared to be an ankh-shaped metal pipe, probably once part of a car's transmission. I backed up, but I wasn't running. I was loaded for bear, holding the barrel of the BB gun in one hand and James Bond in the other.

"Put that pipe down!" Eric's mom yelled.

Eric did not put the pipe down. As a matter of fact, Eric swung the pipe at my temple with everything he had. I dodged the deadly slug, then returned a blow with the BB gun. The handle broke over his head. He stumbled backward, dazed. Eric's big brother, Squanky, lurched toward me from my left side. He was a bully who chased us frequently, especially if we called him by his real name, Ellis. I tossed the broken gun aside and pointed the knife at Ellis's nose.

"Put the knife down, man. Put the knife down, man," Squanky said.

Yeah, right. He wanted me to get rid of the only thing keeping him off me? Thank goodness Squanky had more sense than his brother.

"Squanky, get in this house," his mom demanded.

Squanky retreated with a singeing stare. A. T. pulled me away while I returned Squanky's glare. A. T. ushered me up his stairs into his second-floor apartment. The higher vantage point gave us a fuller view of the fracas. Eric paced in circles, looking up at me in the window.

"Come downstairs, you...punk!" he shouted.

He was choosing his words carefully in his mom's presence. I looked down at him and chuckled. His mom caught my sneer.

"Are you laughing, Rodney? You think this is funny?" she said.

If she could've reached up and yanked me out of that window, she would've. I did think it was kinda funny, but I wasn't going to admit it to her. I mean, why would anyone grab the blade of a knife? She marched into her home, shaking a finger at the sky.

A police car pulled into the parking lot.

Disputes that started in the street were settled in the streets; that was the code. But Eric's mom must've said to herself, "If I can't yank him out of that window, the long arm of the law will." She dramatized the events to the officers. I watched from the window with contempt for her and those like her, the women whose only role was to see me punished.

One officer jotted down notes while the other followed her hand movements, which ended with her finger pointed at me. The officer looked up at me, then waved for me to come out. I folded the 007, and A. T. held the door open.

The officer took down my age, my address, and my side of the story.

"Where's the knife?" he asked. I handed it over to him, thinking I would get it back. I did not. But at least I had my freedom until Mom came home.

"Well, if he grabbed the blade, he got what he deserved," Mom said.

That's what I was saying. A week later, an irregularly sized letter poked out of the mailbox informing me about the court date for Rodney Laney. My run-ins with the law had never landed me in any *real* trouble, other than a soft ass, but this time felt different. This was serious. Bob told Mom she had better get a lawyer.

The lawyer ended up being an old white man. He assessed the paperwork from behind his littered desk, then looked down through his specs to assess me. His scruffy, scraggly attire didn't instill much confidence. Maybe he was like Columbo, I hoped.

I gathered it was the police report he held in his hands.

"Has he ever been in trouble before?" he asked my mom.

"Not with the police...well, not really," Mom said.

"What happened?" the lawyer asked.

I walked him through the events with Eric, and he fixated on one part: whether I had pulled the knife or if Eric had pulled it. He explained that since the knife's blade was more than four fingers or five inches, it wasn't considered a pocketknife.

"Did he grab it and pull it, or did you pull down?" he asked. I could tell he wanted me to say Eric's sliced fingers were his own doing, which was kinda true but not 100 percent. "I'm going to have to talk to the prosecutor, see how far he wants to take this," he concluded.

On the day of my court appearance, Mom took off from work. After circling the block, she found parking, then we hurried toward the courthouse. The top dome of the Passaic County Courthouse resembled an ancient helmet. At the entrance of the building stood six white columns or giant prison bars. We made it in time to be notified that the case had been postponed. Mom loved that, as evidenced by the Laney scowl. The court had randomly summoned us for an appearance, and now it was postponed.

When we went back on the rescheduled date, Mom and Eric's mom, Laura, smoked their cigarettes with their backs to each other while Eric and I studied our shoelaces from opposite ends of the hallway. Eric's slit fingers had long since healed, along with our friendship. In "the Dead End", we were boys, who cracked on each other and laughed, but downtown, we were a plaintiff and a defendant who didn't smile. The courthouse had handcuffed our fellowship.

In the corridor of the municipal building, broken Patersonians leaned against the walls or squatted on the floor. The lucky ones, such as me and Mom that day, sat on the bench. Everyone was waiting to hear if their case had made the docket. I think that's what our lawyer called it. We were waiting for another postponement when our lawyer scrambled over to Mom.

"We're going in front of the judge today," he told her.

He ruffled through his briefcase, searching for his notes. My pulse quickened. Mom looked at me in a way that said it was out of her hands. Her concern caught me off guard and gave me *that* feeling.

It was the same feeling I got when I went home for lunch and she was finalizing my meal: a sizzling bologna sandwich layered with lettuce, tomato, and nongovernment melted cheese on a baked bun; that feeling when she sprinkled chips on my plate and poured an intensely carbonated no-frills soda into a cup, which sparkled underneath my nose and watered my mouth; that feeling she had in her half-opened eyes and full smile when I took a mouthful of her bread.

I couldn't stand myself for making Mom helpless. If I could've manhandled the officers, I would've, but they were real men who had real guns and real bullets. A knife and a gun had gotten me into trouble, but they couldn't get me out of it. Mom patted me on my leg before she stood. I followed her lead.

I thought the legal system would render me innocent. I was naive. I thought the system would call Eric foolish for grabbing the blade of a knife and would send me home free and clear. By the nervousness of my lawyer, I could tell that wasn't the case.

"Let me go and talk to the prosecutor, see if we can work out a plea," the lawyer said.

Eric and his mom had kept their distance. I could tell Mom wanted—no, needed—a cigarette. I put my hand on her shoulder, and for a second, the merry-go-round stilled.

The lawyer returned. "This guy is being a hard-ass; he won't reduce the charges. He's trying to get you the maximum." *The maximum? What the hell is the maximum? Life?* I'd heard about juvie. The guys who survived didn't tell stories about fireworks and birthday cakes.

"We're going to have to go to trial," the lawyer declared.

I needed a cigarette. I leaned my head against the wall. Going to trial meant more money. Money that Mom never complained about but couldn't afford I knew.

"Do you know them?" the lawyer asked. He was referring to Eric and Laura.

"I work with Laura," Mom said.

He turned to me and asked, "And how are you guys?"

"We're cool," I said.

"Mrs. Simmons, you should go talk to her," he told Mom.

Mom marched down the hall toward Laura with a renewed purpose. I don't know what she said, but Laura walked up to a white man in a dark suit holding a tablet. Whatever she said to him made him drop the tablet at his side and glared at her. Mom watched the exchange and then returned.

"She's going to drop the charges," Mom said.

The prosecutor attempted to change Laura's mind, but she dismissed him with a wave of her index finger. Why would he be upset? I guess he really wanted to throw that book at me. I held the door open for Mom and walked through the giant columns feeling like Samson.

In our Pontiac 2000, a breeze entered through my window as I exhaled out of it. Mom loved some Bobby Womack and sang along with "That's the Way I Feel About 'Cha." I knew exactly how Bobby felt.

Discarded.

Dougie Fresh

No going outside and no TV."

After Mom laid down her rules, my bedroom window overlooking the walkway from the parking lot to Haledon Avenue became my only portal to the outside world. The punishing silence made it easy to hear the fellas' footsteps. Whenever I heard them, I pressed against the windowsill and eased open the window. For as long as they would stand, I kept them entertained. I was the original TikTok. I kept them tuned in to a television lineup where I starred in all the programming. I was the only weatherman who had to ask, "How is the weather?"

No matter how entertaining I was, my viewers would inevitably leave. They cited ridiculous excuses for leaving, like the need for food or sleep. "Fine!" I'd exclaim. *Let your biological necessities break up our friendship.*

Once Mom softened restrictions, I was allowed music. I marveled over her new stereo, watching the L-shaped arm scoop up the vinyl, hold it over the turntable for a second, then drop it like it was hot into the perfect position. I observed the needle rotate and then descend with pinpoint accuracy into the groove, inches away from my nose. The music was my only escape. Rene and Angela's "I'll Be Good" made me promise to do the same.

Many of Mom's records came with an instrumental-only version on the flip side, which fertilized my imagination. Inspired to write something, I grabbed my notebook. The need to plagiarize Luther Vandross ended and I wrote my first rap.

The radio station 92 KTU announced that Dougie Fresh and Slick Rick would be live and in concert in East Orange, New Jersey. I asked members of the High-Powered Crew if they wanted to go. The High-Powered Crew was a rap group consisting of Kenny, A. T., Renita, and myself, which had the life span of a summer banana. They declined. *Broke-asses.*

"Your mom's never going to let you go anyway," A. T. said.

First of all, my momma don't run my life…well, actually she does, but that's not the point. A. T. was right, but something as minor as parental consent wasn't going to stop me. The concert was to take place on a Sunday at 5 p.m. My curfew was 8 p.m. That gave me 10,800 seconds—plenty of time to be back in "the Dead End."

"Which bus will get me there?" I asked. A. T. shrugged and gave me an incredulous nod.

On the evening of the concert, I went down to the basement, where I had stashed my concert clothing. I collected my gray sporty Lambeau jacket, took off my everyday sneakers, and slipped into my new joints. I counted out the few dollars I had managed to keep from Mom since she held on to all my earnings. The coast was clear. I stepped off the block in style, headed to a concert that I had no idea how to get to.

I hiked down to the Broadway bus terminal; my first concert was coinciding with my first bus ride. I looked through the leaflets for a bus going to East Orange. The P72 to Newark was the first bus. I hadn't realized I would have to take more than one bus; it's a good thing I had a couple of extra dollars on me.

The bus smelled like cinnamon-flavored doo-doo. I surveyed the passengers looking for someone who was also going to the concert. One familiar commuter stood out from the ragtag strap-hangers. Pop-locking Al sported a turned-to-the-back Kangol hat, a gold tooth, and a blue sporty Lambeau jacket. That cool mofo had Dougie Fresh written all over his face.

"Yo, that jacket is fresh," Al said.

"Thanks," I said.

The compliment meant a lot coming from him—my soon-to-be guide. Seeing Al on the bus reassured me that I had chosen the right bus since he was from East Orange. The ride to EO was longer than I expected. The lack of air conditioning made all of the cinnamon parts of the smell disappear. Al maintained his cool, periodically wiping his brow, picking lint off his jacket, and wiping the front of his shell-toe Adidas sneakers with a napkin he spat into. I brushed off my Pumas, then gazed out the window. Paterson receded from view as we bounced southbound through Clifton.

Al did all of the talking. I did all the listening. He rattled off landmarks for different bus routes. We hopped off the P72 and took another bus, which wouldn't have been in my plan, but Al knew how to shorten the trip. I shadowed him as if my freedom depended on him because it did.

At 5 p.m. the concert hadn't started. I squinted to get a better look at the makeshift stage that sat in the middle of a track-and-field arena fifty yards away. Al scanned the crowd looking for his people. I imagined having the point of view from the stage.

Disenchantment gripped the hip-hop audience because of their distance from the stage. How was Dougie Fresh going to hurdle this obstacle? To alleviate the crowd's growing dissent, he waved his hand, meaning *come down.* With that one gesture of Dougie Fresh's right hand, chaos ensued.

Waves of people charged the fence and tried hopping it. Those who made it over rushed the stage in a mad dash. Those who didn't make it were trampled, caught in an avalanche of bodies. The music was drowned out by screams and shouting. I used my jumping skills to hurdle the fence and rode the wave to the front. The energy went from stale to frantic. A guy leaped onstage and rushed Dougie Fresh.

"My daughter, my daughter!" he screamed.

A burly security guard snatched him off his feet before his arms could reach Dougie's neck.

The concert was already a spectacle without one song having been played. I turned to Al. Slick Rick's "moment I feared" came to mind. It was 6:15, and I had lost Al.

By 6:45, the concert started rocking—right when I had to leave. At 7 p.m. I was back at the bus stop. I'd given myself a half hour to get to the Paterson depot, then I could jog from there and make it home on time.

While I was waiting, a woman passing by took a long pause before speaking: "The buses stop running, sugar. You're gonna have to call your momma."

No outdoors. No TV. No nothing, for the rest of your life. Mom's rant echoed in my mind. Al had failed to mention that the buses stopped running early on Sundays. That seemed a vital part of the tutorial.

I searched the sky for a solution, but even the sun had started to abandon me. *How much could a cab cost?* I wondered. The bus ride was only $1.70; I figured the cab ride couldn't be more than... what, five bucks?

I spotted a cab dropping a passenger off. I hustled over to the car, waving my hands, to inquire about his fare. "Twenty-five dollars," he said. I repeated it out loud. The cab driver's dreadlocks and no-nonsense jawline filled his window. "You wan go?" he asked.

The cost was five times more than what I had in my pocket. "Yeah," I said.

He sucked his tooth and scratched his wiry beard as I slid into the back seat. The cab smelled familiar. "Somebody been smoking ganja, huh?" I joked. My remark got a deadpan look. Cordiality was not his strong suit.

We headed up Central Avenue with his reggae pumping. We passed record shops, bodegas, and chicken joints. The smell of barbecue reminded me that I hadn't eaten since I left home. East Orange's Central Avenue was similar to downtown Paterson.

"We gon take da parkway, mon. Aay tolls me understand," the cabby said. I nodded yes, even though I didn't understand.

It was a day of firsts: first bus ride and first concert. I was about to add another. The cabby interrupted my nail-biting with his frequent glances in the rearview mirror. Right before the freeway entrance, he pulled into a gas station, threw the car in park, then turned over his shoulder.

"I need gus, so Imma need da money now," the cabby said.

My plan hadn't incorporated a gas stop. "Uh, I don't have the money now, but my mom will pay you when we get there," I told him.

"So you don't have any money on you?"

"I only have five dollars."

"Gib it."

When he exited the cab, I saw all of him. He was six feet tall— *good lord*. He jogged inside the gas station with a Carl Lewis stride.

I assumed he was Jamaican, but his sprint back made me think he was part Nigerian. I'd picked the *wrong motha.*

Potholes and the prison welcomed me back to downtown Paterson. He silenced the music as if to keep focus. His rearview-mirror scrutiny intensified as we motored through the streets. His Jamaican sixth sense must've kicked in because he stopped coming to complete stops and began rolling through stops signs. I directed him past school twenty-eight, up Temple Hill, and toward Lilly Street—a dark, dead-end street adjacent to the block of freedom.

"Uh…right here is good," I said.

Outrunning this Olympian wasn't going to work. And he wouldn't hesitate to deliver Rastafarian justice. He parked underneath the only functioning streetlamp. I reviewed my plan.

"You better not tink but doin' anyting stupid," the cabby said. *Too late for that.*

My plan was to run through this elderly woman's yard and hop over the stone wall that separated her yard from the Hobsons' backyard. For the plan to work, I needed two dogs to be housed: the old lady's Doberman Pinscher and the Hobsons' German shepherd, named Bull. Bull was known for chasing and biting anyone who was running, and he loved jumping on cars.

I reached for the car handle. Before I could open it, the cabby grabbed my arm.

"I'm going to get your money," I said.

"Imma need some collateral," the cabby said.

"I don't have any collat—"

He snatched my glasses midsentence. The shock to my vision caused me to blink incessantly. The Rasta blurred.

"When you come back wit de money, I'll give dem back," he said.

My extreme nearsightedness prevented any chance of seeing the guard dogs. I fumbled toward the gate, squinting to see the latch. When it came into focus, I could clearly see it was padlocked. The gig was up.

I heaved myself over the fence. *Boom!* The cab door slammed shut. The Rastafarian was on the loose. I ran up the side of the house, guided by instinct and intuition. Keys jingled, and they were closing in on me. I was running faster than my vision, which is why I slammed into a concrete wall. I kept my footing because I didn't have time to fall. I scaled the wall, looked down into a fuzzy abyss, then leaped. I'd jumped off that wall plenty of times and cleared the shrubbery from memory. I tore down the Hobsons' driveway and saw a fuzzy but familiar body.

A. T. saw me hauling ass out of the backyard and started running with me. No questions asked. We ran through the parking lot, past A. T.'s apartment. I'd planned to keep running past my house and down the steps, but my door swung open and Mom stepped out.

"Rodney?" she said. I broke stride coming to a wild stop. A. T. kept truckin'.

I bent over, gasping for air, squinting for a crazed Jamaican. Mom searched the hill, looking to see who I was running from.

"Where are your glasses?" she asked.

"I took them off. I didn't want to break them."

She held me in place with her skeptical gaze. "Well, come in and eat," she said.

That was music to my ears.

Discarded.

Crab

Thousands of Kennedy students paraded up Preakness Avenue toward an X-shaped building. Teachers joked privately that the X marked the target for a bomb. I kept pace with A. T., who had been a knight for two years. Although he didn't say it, I could tell he didn't want to be seen with a freshman, lest he has to endure the hazing as well. Once we got close to the high school, A. T. ditched me for other juniors. I was a knight without a shield.

Our high school, JFK, never received the notoriety of its rival high school, Eastside, whose delinquency was the subject of the movie *Lean on Me*. Its principal, Joe Clark, a bat- and bullhorn-toting authoritarian, was played by Morgan Freeman. Kennedy's violence wasn't as well-known as Eastside's, and that's why it had something to prove.

There weren't as many gangs in Paterson in the 1980s as there were in, say, Chicago or Los Angeles. We had posses—cliques of ruffians who differentiated themselves by their block. There were the Main, the Northside, the CCP projects, the Grand Street projects, Union Avenue, North Third, North Fourth, and more. All the posses crossed each other in the hallways of the three-story high school building. Freshmen who were part of a posse were protected. The fiercest protection came from your family. Loners, like me, were vulnerable.

Loading and unloading Bob's truck over the summer had paid off. I had saved enough money to replace my snatched glasses with expensive designer frames. In the hallways, I saw clearly the attention my Cazals brought. High school was a'aight.

The day after the first day of school, a Wednesday, A. T. and I stopped by Roger's before the thirty-minute hike to Kennedy. While I was walking up North Fourth street, someone snatched my Cazals. The blurry thief cut out of sight before my vision settled. *What is with these mofos and my glasses?*

Thanks to A. T.'s twenty-twenty vision, he recognized the thief: a guy named Crab. The name befit him. He was the oldest of three brothers, which meant I couldn't get my Cazals back on my own.

Luckily, I had help: a guy Aunt Mildred had started dating Willis, a linebacker who looked as if he only ate ham-hocks and beef shoulders. He played for the New York Giants. If I had to guess, I'd say his career must've spanned a three-day weekend. Aunt Mildred had heard what happened and sent Willis to my defense.

How Willis squeezed his body behind the wheel of Aunt Mildred's Fiero was worthy of a segment on *That's Incredible!* He could steer the wheel with his pecs. Invigorated, I peered out the window, looking for Mr. Crustacean. We pulled up to a drug-dealing corner. Emboldened by the hulking beast at my side, I hopped out.

"Y'all see Crab?" I asked. The posse looked past me toward the driver, then shook their heads no. I punched my palm, then used my middle finger to push my taped-up glasses back to the brim of my nose to complete the tough academic look. We peeled off, leaving them wondering why Crab's tutor was looking for him.

We searched the Main, the Northside, the CCP projects, the Grand Street projects, Union Ave, North Third, and North Fourth, then around school twelve and back to Roger's. Crab had sub-merged, and who knew how long he would lie low? I thanked Willis and watched him go into swami mode and contort himself before driving down Haledon Avenue.

That Friday, our small posse searched the corners, avenues, and alleyways for the thief, led by my cousin Rocky. Being on foot gave us a better vantage point, putting us closer to the rats, snakes, and crabs.

"There he is," someone finally said.

My heart fluttered. Crab was leaning against the railing of a staircase between two houses, calm and untroubled as we closed in. The reasons for his equanimity revealed themselves one by one. By the time we reached him, his posse had assembled as if they had been waiting on us. Not only did they outnumber us, but we had invaded their block. Retreating wasn't an option. We disregarded rationality the way that punk had disregarded me when he snatched my dignity. I anxiously waited to see Rocky crack him open.

"My cousin said you stole his Cazals?" Rocky said.

"I didn't steal nobody's Cazals," Crab said.

"Yes, you did," I said.

Demolish this punk, Rocky. Rocky looked at me.

"Well, it's your word against his. You know how we settle this in the streets," Rocky said.

I nodded *yeah.* No idea.

"You're going to have to shoot a fair one," Rocky said.

Damn. Why can't he just give my shit back?

"You want to fight him?" Rocky asked.

Why would he ask me that in front of everybody? *Not really. I thought that was your job. We should've had a roundtable discussion about this earlier.* Both posses waited for a response.

"Yeah," I said.

Clapping and "hooraying" replaced the wolf stares given by both camps. I rolled up my sleeves and handed Rocky my glasses and my ability to see clearly. I backed up as Crab came down to meet me at street level. He removed his hoodie and moved his head laterally, a boxer warming up. Each step I took gave momentum to the next—small victories in of themselves. We squared off, sizing each other up. The pressure to take a swing caused me to throw a hook, which landed me in a feeling of weightlessness as if I were airborne. Crab had scooped my legs and driven me into the concrete. *Yep. Slammed again.*

I lay on the sidewalk, shattered to pieces. Crab's blurred image stood over me, but he was staring at Rocky.

"Any more questions?" Crab asked.

"Yeah, I got one," Rocky said. Both sides waited for his question.

"Where you learn to slam like that?" Rocky said.

His retort unified both sides in laughter. As if landing on my back weren't enough, I also got stabbed in it. *Thanks a lot, family.*

I dusted myself off, put on my backup glasses, and took a solemn walk home. Mom greeted me at the door, relieved and curious: "Did you get your glasses back? What happened? Did you find him?" I shook my head and went to my room and didn't bother turning on the light.

Saturday morning, I woke up feeling more alone than I'd ever felt in my life. I had never met anyone with my last name. I went into the living room, pulled the yellow pages from underneath the coffee table, and flipped through the pages of the phone book, tracing my finger down the pages of the "L" section. Nothing. Not one single Laney in the Paterson white pages.

Discarded.

Michelle

The one person who didn't mind the sudden rash of eyewear snatchings was my optometrist. Dr. Cohn's spearmint-flavored breath seeped up my nose while he burned my retina with his mini flashlight. After he murmured approvingly, he eased my chin and forehead against a machine that resembled hi-tech binoculars. He spun the wheel of prescriptions, and the test part of the eye exam began.

"Is this better, worse, or about the same?" Dr. Cohn asked.

I detested eye exams because of my failure rate.

"How 'bout this one? Better or worse?" Dr. Cohn said.

"The same," I said.

I was only there because of Mom's resolution to my problem. Her solution involved an actual solution, plus a heating unit and enzymatic protein tablets. We left the office with all the necessities for my first pair of contact lenses.

The next day, Michelle glimpsed the new look as I left Roger's, and she smiled, which made me pause for the cause. She had the attributes I wanted in a female: reserved, unpopular, and interested in me—the latter being the most crucial. Her nurturing lips, curvy hips, and double Ds made it easy to reciprocate. She lived a few houses away from Roger's on North Fourth street in a house where everybody and their momma hung out. I had to get her to the pit—our basement—if I wanted intimacy.

I coaxed her down into our basement, guided her through the darkness, and sat her up on the washing machine. I titillated her by caressing her ears, cheeks, and neck, but I must've been moving too slowly. She wrapped her legs around my waist and yanked me by the back of my head, then planted her juicy lips on my face. Our first kiss was breathtaking. Not because it was miraculous but because I couldn't breathe.

The first fifteen minutes, I was able to stay afloat, but the in last fifteen, I started drowning in slobber. Every time I tried backing out of the kiss, she clutched the back of my head, holding me in her vice grip. I opened my eyes and watched her marinate my mouth with her scent. *A quiet girl, my ass.*

Two hours later—when the kiss ended—my contacts had dried out and were stuck to my eyeballs. She had sucked the moisture from my body. All the fluids that had once been in my body had seeped into my shirt. Footsteps overhead meant Mom had arrived, my cue to get Michelle back home. She collected herself while I considered throwing my shirt in the dryer. On the way back, she wanted to know if she could ever be my girlfriend.

As long as we never have to kiss again, I thought.

Discarded.

Rebellion

The corner store was a cornerstone of a neighborhood. Each minimart had its own flavor, depending on the ethnicity of the owner and its location. The Clinton and North Sixth store was known for craps games, which took place at the side of the building. A. T. and I approached the store one day, concealing our concern over the posse on the corner. Friendliness was reserved for the familiar, and we were strangers.

As we left the store, Lance, a skinny dude with a knack for being annoying, made his presence known. I knew him from school twelve. He examined me, looking for the slightest imperfection in my gear, face, or sneakers, searching for anything to crack on. I ran through my list of comebacks, ready to return fire. He was as bony as those Ethiopians in the commercials who needed food. *You big for-a-dollar-a-day-save-an-Ethiopian-looking....*

I didn't know how the posse was going to react to my bust, so it would be a hit-and-move game of dozens. Before Lance could take his jab, a car screeched to a halt. Two white uniformed police officers hopped out of their cruiser.

"Here come the overseers," someone shouted.

Dice banged against the wall. If they landed on seven or eleven, no one knew. All eyes, even the snake eyes, were on the officers. No one ran. Everyone and everything halted. The authorities ordered the posse to clear the block.

"Let's skedaddle," I said. A. T. was already skedaddling. The dice were picked up as the players complied with the orders.

All except Lance. "Why?" he asked.

The question ceased the dispersion. Lance stood alone as the policemen closed in on him, with their nightsticks swaying at their sides.

"Get on the ground," the police ordered.

"Why do I have to get on the ground?" Lance said.

It seemed a reasonable question to me. I mean, Paterson's streets weren't the most sanitary places to be lying on. One of the cops grabbed Lance. Although Lance didn't resist, the officer still plowed him into the street. His face smacked the blacktop, reminiscent of a whip cracking a bareback. I winced in pain.

"You feel like a man now?" Lance said.

The other cop rushed over and kneeled on Lance's frail shoulder blade with his gun, his bulletproof vest, his handcuffs, his ammunition, all of his two-hundred-pound body, and his metal badge.

"Leave him alone!" a female pleaded.

"Get off me," Lance said.

The boys in blue yanked Lance off the ground, then shoved him in the back of the squad car. Blood trickled from his temple down his scraped cheek. They drove off with him as we all stood by and watched.

"Another day in the hood," A. T. said.

Discarded.

Mr. Sherman

While sitting in Mr. Hazuda's freshman class, I drew a bearded man's face on the body of a donkey and wrote "Mr. Sherman" underneath it. I passed the drawing around class and reveled in the laughter. Mr. Sherman was an asshole because he was good at his job: terrorizing students.

A messenger tapped on the open door of Mr. Hazuda's class, saying, "Mr. Sherman wants to see Rodney Laney." A round of "oohs" and "aahs" ushered me to the doorway, where my escort awaited.

"Somebody take good notes for me," I said. *Damn, I almost got away with it.*

Mr. Sherman leaned over his desk, bringing his salt-and-pepper beard within two inches of my nose, yelling at me as if he wanted to fight. Behind all that hot nicotine-scented breath was a demand to know why I had cut his class. I folded my arms and looked in the corner, considering how much a yawn would raise his blood pressure. I ignored him until he threatened to call Mom.

"She doesn't care. Call her," I said.

"We'll see about that. If I see you in here again, you'll be suspended. Get out of here."

I smirked, then pimp-walked out of his office and through the building without an iota of concern. Once I turned the corner, I straightened up and began gnawing my fingernails. I had to inter-cept that call.

When the school called, which wasn't often, I knew by the way Mom would answer: "This is she. Uh-hm, OK. Can you hold on a minute? Tasha, go get me a cigarette." Tasha would bring her a cigarette, then give me an "I wouldn't want to be you" head nod. Smoking cigarettes calmed Mom's nerves and rattled mine. They were definitely bad for my health.

"Tasha, bring me another cigarette," Mom called that evening. Damn, it was Mr. Sherman. I stood in the living room, hanging on to every word of the conversation. If it was a one-cigarette phone call, I might get away with confinement to the porch or to the house. "Uh-huh. No, I was not aware of that. OK. Hold on a sec-ond, please. Tasha, bring me another cigarette."

Another cigarette? My immediate future was looking dismal. I was looking at hard time in isolation, or worse, she might even consider the cord. I never talked back to Mom; her authority went mostly uncontested. I listened and ducked when necessary. But I was in high school now and too old for whoopings. I didn't dare say this to my thirty-four-year-old mom, but how long would I allow this to go on?

Mom hung up the phone and came for me. She cornered me in the kitchen with my back against the closet as she unleashed an epic hissy fit. Then she stopped as if someone had hit her mute button. Mom had noticed something that created the deepest Laney scowl I ever saw.

"You balling up at me? You balling up at me?" Mom said.

My fists were balled up.

"You want to hit me! Just 'cause you taller than me?" Mom said.

I unballed my fists.

"Go ahead and try it," Mom said.

I held up both my open hands. *Don't shoot.* She staggered out of the kitchen and slammed her bedroom door.

On my bed, I observed my fists as if it were the first time I'd ever seen them. *How'd you get like that?* It was as if my body had a mind of its own.

Discarded.

Cheeba

A long pull from the joint made it flare in the dark garage, illuminating A. T.'s face as he watched his student take his first toke. Smoke hit my lungs, causing a burst of convulsions from my body as it rejected it. My snorts and squeals sounded similar to hogs mating. A. T. laughed.

"Your eyeballs damn near came out their sockets," he said. "You have to hold the smoke in."

The smoke didn't want to be held in. I looked at A. T. with watery eyes, nodded, and continued coughing. Why anyone would purposely suck on smoke to get high was baffling.

A. T. had convinced me to cut school, so we were holed up in someone's garage. I wasn't comfortable in the garage at 11 a.m.; it reminded me too much of a basement—the kind of basement that cops raid. As we emerged from the darkness, reality slowed to the ideal pace. I held my hand to shield my eyes from the sun's brilliance. Herds of clouds stampeded through the sky. Everything was all goody-goody in the hoody-hoody.

"Wow, it's still daytime," I said.

"You high?" A. T. asked.

"I think so."

My fascination with the sky transitioned into an awareness that cutting school was a terrible idea. My thoughts became erratic and suspicious: Mr. Sherman knew we had cut school and was already calling my mother. He couldn't know that already. Could he? I howled with laughter. *I'm so silly. What time is it? I'm hungry.*

We walked from North Seventh Street to the historical landmark responsible for Paterson's existence. Mother Nature had blessed us with the best show in town: the Paterson Great Falls. Although I'd seen the seventy-seven-foot drop dozens of times, I had never seen it like this. I was trapped in my own amazement. A footbridge hovered over the cliffs and connected one side of the park to the other. I set one foot on the bridge, and my heart pounded my eardrums as I watched the rapids break over the precipice. I took another step, and the bridge wobbled—at least it did in my mind. I looked back to see if A. T. was coming, but he was sitting on the bench, sparking another blunt. I backed off the bridge. The thought of falling alone was sobering.

One day not long after the day we cut school, the smell of sess lured me into the third-floor bathroom in the west wing of Kennedy. A guy stood at the entrance, the bathroom's bouncer. I expected a pat-down, but he took a pull from a blunt and nodded *OK*. He kicked wet paper towels against the door to create a seal. Exhalations of ganja made the john hazy and softened the light. The first two stalls were filled with smokers. The third stall was filled with an unholy amount of the Devil's dung.

Wendell, my old classmate, was in a cipher, a circular huddle, waiting for his turn to puff. I gave him a pound while eyeing the blunt. I had never smoked in school before, and up until then hadn't considered it, but there's a first time for everything.

I whizzed and washed my hands, then dried them on my pant legs because the bouncer had used all the paper towels on the door. Wendell hit the blunt before raising it toward me, gesturing for me to take it. His fat lips had made the joint extra soggy, which initially deterred me.

"Hit it," Wendell said.

One hit couldn't hurt. I pinched the wet blunt between my fingers, careful to get his saliva on my fingers and not on my lips.

Suddenly someone locked the bathroom door *from the outside.*

"They locked us in," the bouncer said.

A security guard spoke into his walkie-talkie: "We've got them locked in."

The bouncer yanked the door. I put the blunt back in Wendell's hand and wiped his spit off my fingers.

"Man, I got two strikes already, homey," he said.

No surprise there. A third strike meant expulsion for him and goodbye to the school year. He dipped into a stall as someone slid the bathroom door's deadbolt back. When the security guard opened the door, the smoke fanned back into our faces, clearing the way for Mrs. Chase.

The itty-bitty woman would patrol the hallways like a caffeinated Yorkie, looking for wrongdoers. She despised weed smokers, giving them harsh penalties. She was the vice president—beloved by some, detested by others. She was *the* authority figure. Your outcome was bleak when you had to face Mrs. Chase.

"Who was smoking in here?" she asked. Three guards followed her, and the last one stood where the bouncer had been. Avoiding her gaze meant staring at the ceiling as she marched beneath our chins. A guard cleared the stalls. He grimaced at the anal cake in stall three before opening the stall where Wendell was hiding.

Mrs. Chase began her inspection, looking for dilated pupils and smelling for weed breath.

"If no one steps up, all of you are going to get suspended," she said.

The bell rang; now I'd have to explain why I didn't return to class. And if I didn't get to my next class before attendance was taken, I was guaranteed another trip to see Mr. Sherman. No one stepped forward.

"Everyone put out their fingertips," Mrs. Chase said.

Our fingertips? Was she looking for burnt fingers? She started taking whiffs of everyone's blunt holder: their thumb and index finger. I started to smell mine to see if that soggy blunt had left trace evidence but caught myself. That would've been a giveaway.

After a clean sniff, "You're free to go," Mrs. Chase said. After a dirty whiff: "Stand over there." The dirty fingers stood by security. That nose was coming for Mr. Two Strikes and me. Wendell had a plan that he executed while in that stall. Later he would tell me that he'd stuck his fingers up his ass.

Mrs. Chase eyed Wendell, smirking as if his guilt were a foregone conclusion. She snatched his hand, pulling his fingers toward her flared nostrils.

"Goddamn!" she said. She shoved his hands aside in disgust. Wendell kept his composure.

"Stand over there by security," Mrs. Chase said. "Wash your hands first."

The inspection ended due to her devastated olfactory sense. The rest of us left peacefully. I made it to my next class before the teacher finished taking attendance. I resolved to never smoke in school again.

Wendell avoided suspension. How could she have suspended him for foul fingers? Everyone knows the bathroom is where shit happens.

Discarded.

Sherice

On a warm September afternoon during my sophomore year, we piled into Kennedy's auditorium for a quasi pep rally. At least space was a dedicated auditorium and didn't have the identity crisis of school twelve's cafe-gym-atorium. The chairs automatically folded when you stood up; when we all stood up in unison, it sounded like thunder and made applause sound like lightning.

There were nine hundred knights in a room built for eight hundred. Paper balls popped the noggins of those stupid enough to sit up front. Summer's energy had held fast to our spirits, and the restlessness was apparent. Cooping us up in a mandatory assembly during a golden autumn afternoon was disrespectful to Mother Nature and didn't sit well with me. While checking out the curves on the student body, I noticed there were only two security guards: one posted at the far-right corner and the other at the left. The middle aisle went unguarded. I started plotting.

The production had stalled, and the delay instigated the audience's contempt. Throats started clearing as some of the knights prepped their windpipes, ready to boo. It was amateur night at the Apollo, and "The Sandman" was on deck. The theater held eight hundred students, but could it contain them? I doubted it.

"Welcome, class of eighty-seven," Mrs. Chase announced.

That was smart. If anyone but the vice president had stepped onto the stage, they surely would've been booed, but no one would heckle Mrs. Chase. I paid little attention to the Yorkie and slid to the edge of my seat, observing the guards. Then Mrs. Chase surprised me by saying a name that made me slide back in my seat with one thought: *They better not boo her.* The girl approached the microphone and cleared her throat.

Mietta sang. I hadn't heard her voice in years, ever since that last day we'd been together in Mrs. Mary's apartment.

After singing, she hummed this melodious moan that flooded my forearms with goosebumps. It was the type of sound you make when something feels so, so, so damn good. Her gospel voice took me back to church and replaced my anxiety with serenity. When she struck her final note, the knights rose. Thunder and lightning filled the auditorium. It was the perfect storm.

Giving Mietta props and getting reacquainted had to wait, as finding her afterward proved impossible. I hummed down Totowa Avenue, over to Kearney Street, along Union Avenue, and up Belmont Avenue until I reached North Seventh street on what was the most harmonious day of the fall.

The next day was the first full day of classes. Foot traffic filled the hallways. The new knights clustered the hallways, disoriented while looking for room numbers. The freshmen sidestepped the seniors, for good reason.

Wallace and Brandon, two football players, saw a freshman reading his schedule, paying little attention to the two brutes. Not a good idea. Wallace smacked him in the nuts and shouted, "Open nuts!" The freshman doubled over, grimacing as his schedule drifted to the floor. I covered my scrotum with my Spanish book and kept looking for my classroom.

Spanish II was already my favorite class because it was the last one of the day. The students were looking at quizzes in their hands with contempt. Making my way toward the back, I spotted the only person who could answer my question: Where had Mietta learned to sing so passionately? *Por suerte*, luckily, the seat behind Mietta was unoccupied.

"*Hola, gran cantante*," I said.

"*Hola, gracias.*"

Mietta scanned the quiz.

"Who gives a quiz on the first day?" I asked her. "I should bounce. How do you say 'he left' in Spanish?"

"*Se fue.* You leaving?"

"I would if you weren't here. "

I couldn't see Mietta's expression from the back, but she had to be smiling.

"I'll stay here forever. How you say 'forever'?" I said.

"*Para siempre.*"

Mrs. Garcia looked our way.

"We should probably take our quiz," Mietta said.

I postponed my examination of Mietta until after I failed the Spanish test.

After weeks of whispering over Mietta's shoulder, we became more than *amigos*. I asked Mietta out, hoping to begin where we left off, especially since now I knew what "doing it" meant. I walked her home to the Brook-Sloate projects. She resided deep inside the 241-unit low-rise housing complex. The buildings were spread over twenty-three acres and provided dozens of places to get ambushed.

I feared the "Five-O" more than the crews leaning on their cars. When the police arrived, it was usually to make sure no hanky-panky was taking place. Mietta's mom, Officer Stancil, patrolled the area and made surprise check-ins.

In her apartment, we sat on the sofa, taking advantage of Mietta's little sister's absence. The lovey-dovey session turned into a sticky situation. Wrapped up in the moment, I didn't hear the police cruiser pull up. A key was inserted into the doorknob, and Mietta hopped up and skedaddled with her ankles handcuffed by her panties. Her gun-toting mother opened the door, looking for probable cause. I straightened my shirt and smiled as if I didn't have an erection. Officer Stancil paused in the doorway when she caught a glimpse of me. Her keys sounded like a gunshot when they landed on the table.

"What's your name again?" Officer Stancil asked.

"Rodney."

"Where's Mietta?"

Pulling her panties up, I thought. "She went in the back," I said.

Mietta's return interrupted the interrogation and garnered a look from her mom, signaling her surprise at my presence. I took the cue. Her badge, bra, and nightstick had an emasculating effect on what was in my jeans. I felt comfortable enough to stand without revealing any bulges or my intentions.

"Don't leave on my account," Officer Stancil said. I thanked her for her kindness, hugged her daughter, and bounced.

"*Yo queria mas*" became my favorite expression from Spanish class because I wanted more. Mietta lived in the church, working overtime singing for the Lord. Jesus infringed on our time. The classroom and the short walk home were the only opportunities I had to spend with her, and they left me wanting.

When Mietta missed class one Monday, it meant three days without seeing her. And although it seemed irrational, the thought of never seeing her again flickered in my mind. I knew she wouldn't cut class and risk a trip to Mr. Sherman's office. Perhaps she was sick?

Only a few perceptive classmates knew we were dating since we didn't flaunt our relationship. Sandra Blair was observant.

"How's Mietta doing?" Sandra said.

"I'm not sure, to be honest," I said.

"Did she go home because of her pregnancy?"

"Pregnancy!" I laughed at the odd remark.

"She's pregnant, right?" Sandra continued.

"Hell nah," I smirked at Sandra's nonsense. No way.

That day after school, my favorite tune, "Outstanding" by the Gap Band, made me two-step and sway in the kitchen. Since Mom and Tasha weren't around, I cranked the radio and sang along.

I boogied over to the Wonder Bread, did the Wop while spreading peanut butter and jelly, and—after taking a hearty mouthful—I started doing the Mietta hum. I did the George Jefferson slide over to the telephone and dialed to the beat.

Mom and Tasha hadn't met Mietta since we'd rekindled our relationship, but it was time. The innovative cordless phone freed me to roam the entire apartment, all four hundred square feet. Mietta answered.

"Sherice," I said.

I called her by her middle name since few knew it, and no one used it. It made me feel as if I knew her better than anyone else.

"You a'aight? I missed you in Spanish class today," I told her.

"I'm fine."

The small talk gave way to the looming absurdity coiled in the back of my mind.

"Guess what?" I asked.

"What?"

"People made up all kinds of reasons for you missing class. Sandra even asked me if you was pregnant. Crazy."

I roamed into my room. Lisa Lisa's "I Wonder If I Take You Home" played over the silence.

"I am pregnant," she said.

Uncle Butch had once shown us pictures of a man hit and pinned by a subway car. He said they call a priest in those situations because once they remove the train, the person's internal organs collapse, and he dies.

Mietta had removed my train.

The phone fell onto the carpet and rested at my feet. It slipped from my grasp like reality had.

"Hello? Hello? Rodney, are you there?... Are you there?" Mietta asked.

Her voice cleared the fog. I bent over.

"Are you there?" Mietta repeated.

I am here, I thought. But I didn't want to be. I only wanted to be *there*, with her.

"I need to see you," I declared.

I dumped the sandwich in the trash, killed the radio, then headed to Mietta's.

Holy shit! Mietta was freaking pregnant. During the three months of our relationship, we had fooled around, but the most I'd achieved was what Alfie called "fish fingers." *Who was the father?*

What am I going to do? What are we going to do? All my questions were suppressed by my need to hold her. I ran, jogged, speed-walked, and ran some more until I reached my watery-eyed girlfriend on her porch. Tears sprung from the corners of my eyes as I hugged her as tight as I could. The life in her belly filled the emptiness in mine.

Mietta's pregnancy had started before our relationship. Apparently, there had been some hanky-panky in the pulpit. I think she expected me to flip out when she told me she was giving the baby's father another shot, but what good would flipping out do? My tantrum days were over.

Monday arrived without Mietta.

Ella se fue, para siempre. She had left for good.

Discarded.

"We Need a Plan"

I bobbed up and down on the swishy mattress, sending slow-motion ripples from the foot of the bed to the headboard. The waterbed occupied most of Supreme's bedroom. I wondered how the youngest boy in a family of seven had managed to have a room to himself. Supreme played his Atari 2600, oblivious to my backstroke that was worthy of the Olympics. I concluded two things after winning my heat: Supreme had to be his dad's favorite, and weed was the bomb diggity.

Mr. Griffin, Supreme's dad, owned a two-family home on the dead-end part of Lily Street—the same street I hopped a cab. Once Mr. Griffin arrived, Supreme vanished—well, the name did. Only the names Mr. Griffin bestowed were used in his house. He didn't give a damn about Supreme's "righteousness." He called him Danny. And Danny called him Dad, every chance he got. At least in my mind.

"Heads up!" Barbara said.

The alert meant Dad was coming. A frenzy in Supreme's room followed the call. Murk, Supreme's older brother, directed the action. A. T., Supreme, and two girls named Sheila and Barbara followed his command to clear the rolling papers, blunts, and beer bottles. Murk kept one eye out the window and one on the cleanup.

The exterior door opened, sending the family's dog, Rex, barking and running to the door.

Mr. Griffin stroked Rex under his throat, then scanned the room, checking us out. His head tilted to the side as he examined me, probably wondering why I looked petrified.

Our "party" had started hours earlier.

At first, my lungs had tingled a bit, then a burning sensation in my chest followed as I held in the smoke from a joint.

"Hold it...hold it," Murk said.

I rocked back and forth, tapping my foot, fighting my biological urge to breathe. My lungs won the battle and ejected smoke from my nose, mouth, and rectum. The half lung I hacked up incited laughter. Supreme gestured for me to pass the spliff. I recouped and took another hit, saying: "I'm a hitter, not a quitter."

No matter how aloof weed smokers appear, they maintain clarity on two things: who's got the blunt and how many hits they've taken. Two was the limit for us. Murk held everyone's attention as he expounded his ganja-inspired life philosophy. No one gave a damn about what he was talking about, only that he had already taken one hit. As he illustrated with the blunt, the fire between his fingers started zigzagging in slow motion, leaving a streak resembling Halley's Comet. *Is anyone else seeing this?* I wondered.

Murk's philosophy started making sense—a clear sign I was high. It made more than sense; it was genius. Who knew nappy-headed Murk was W. E. B. Dubois reincarnated? My inner voice amplified. *What time is it? It feels late. I'm high. Real, real high. Am I saying this out loud? Can they hear my thoughts? What time is it? Is he ever going to pass the blunt?*

When it was my turn to hit the spliff again, I waved it off, saying: "Nah."

"You high already?" Murk said.

"No. Yes. Hell, yeah. What time is it?"

I heard the embers in the joint crackling. The smoke fell from Murk's nostrils and rolled down his shirt, making him resemble a fired-up Amiri Baraka. I started giggling. Listening to myself laugh made me laugh harder, starting a cycle that spiraled and spread until we all were cracking up. We lost our minds...and sense of time. Barbara, their cousin who lived upstairs, rumbled down the steps and banged on the door.

"Heads up!" she shouted.

Murk ran to the window. "Dad's home early," he announced.

Cleanup and evacuate mode started. They dumped ashtrays, lit incense, and shut off the music. Supreme waved the burning incense as he scuttled through the living room and dining room, leaving a trail of zigzagging smoke. I wanted to bolt through the back door, but all I could do was watch the frenzy from my chair. I was stuck.

"I can't move," I said.

No one heard me. The cover-up continued while Murk stood behind the curtain. I strained to unfreeze myself.

"Rodney, get up," Murk said.

"I'm serious. I can't move," I said.

Rex's barking startled me within my paralysis. Mr. Griffin was at the front door, while A. T. and Sheila were snaking out the back. I focused on my hands, trying to will them into action. Nothing. I moved my attention to my legs. *Come on, Rodney, you can do this!*

The door opened. Mr. Griffin's jacket lay over his shoulders as he surveyed his family. Then his eyes landed on me. His look asked, *Why is the kid sweating?* Because this kid had overcome paralysis in the nick of time. I eased my way between him and Rex on the way out. "Good morning, Mr. Griffin," I said.

No more prerolled joints for me, I thought. I doubted that was the only sess we smoked. *It had to have been laced with something else,* I thought. We changed our supplier to a Jamaican dude named Patrick. All of our dealings took place in his backyard or in his basement. Pat was a straight-up guy unless he was passing through his basement door when he had to crouch. There wasn't any reason for me to think he would harm us.

When we went to buy from Pat the first time, he invited us to partake in his new stock. In the rear corner of his basement sat a brick room with one door, perfect for smoking. The lot of us—Junnie, A. T., and myself—were crammed into the mausoleum. A shoe-box-size window cast light on a couch, rickety chairs, and paint-bucket stools. The metal-bladed fan hummed as it circulated the smell of damp sess.

Murk tapped on the door and stood in the doorway, deciding if he would join us. I didn't think he would stay since he never hung with us young bucks. Pat's sess must've persuaded him.

The lit ends of several blunts cut through the thickening smog. Murk started philosophizing to anyone who listened, which was no one. Everyone fell into their own trance, which is why no one noticed Pat's disappearance.

A. T. raised the spliff to his lips, to everyone's alarm.

"You already had two hits. Pass that." Junnie said.

"Shhhh," Murk said.

A scuffle right outside the door silenced us. The fan hummed. A. T. took a third hit off the blunt. A crack and a thump made all of us hold our breath. It was the familiar sound of a body hitting the ground. Someone on the other side of that door had gotten knocked out. Where was Pat?

"Lock the door," Murk said.

Junnie latched the door, hoping to keep the assailants locked out. But by doing so, he'd sealed us in. The tiny window offered no chance of escape. My shoulder blades were pressed against the stone wall, while my attention was pressed on the doorknob. Waiting for it to turn.

"Somebody got Pat," Junnie mouthed.

"We need a plan," Murk whispered.

A plan? I thought. *What are we, the damn A-Team?* Junnie whipped out his 007, ready to poke whoever came through the door. A. T. stood on a bucket, trying to squeeze through that teeny-tiny window. Physics definitely wasn't his strong suit.

With no other choice, we manned up and formed a semicircle around the door. Murk goaded Junnie to open the door while we crouched and braced for what was on the other side. The 007 wasn't enough protection for Junnie, so he grabbed a chair and held it like a lion tamer. He stuck the tip of the blade under the latch and raised it. His jumpiness caused the latch to rise and fall back in place. A. T. stepped off the bucket, giving up on the impossible. I squared up to face whoever was coming. The latch popped out of the ring, and someone kicked the door open, saying, "I got you mafuckers."

Patrick jumped through, sporting a big everything-will-be-all-right smile, laughing his ass off.

Between Murk's "We need a plan," Junnie's lion tamer, and A. T.'s attempt to alter reality, I couldn't tell you which one made me laugh the hardest.

"It ain't that funny," Murk said.

It was to me, Mr. "We Need a Plan." Even tough guys could get punked, I saw.

Discarded.

The Oak Tree

The roots of an oak tree had raised a section of the concrete sidewalk at the corner of North Seventh and Lily, often tripping up local pedestrians. One of the concrete slabs jutted up at an angle, making it a ramp. Before we'd gotten too cool to ride bikes, the ramp would catapult us in the air, high enough to high-five the leaves. We gave the tree its proper respect, lest we stumble.

One day a commotion near the oak quickened A. T.'s and my pace as we rounded the corner. At the center of the activity was Antney, Supreme's brother. Barbara was there sobbing, then she rapidly pounded the bark of the tree with her fist.

"He's going to get his!" Barbara declared.

"What happened?" A. T. asked.

In between the cussing and crying, we learned that Supreme's older brother had been fighting a guy named Larry Peterkin. Mr. Griffin had stepped in to break it up, apparently in a way that enraged Larry.

Larry left and returned with an aluminum bat, which he used to strike Mr. Griffin on his crown. Police cruisers remained behind after the ambulance rushed Supreme's father to the hospital. His blood seeped through the cracked sidewalk, down to the roots of the oak tree.

A war between the Griffins and Peterkins was looming, and in the words of Murk, they needed a plan. My plan started with finding Supreme. A. T. and I ran to the "Dead End" and hopped down the steps leading to Eric's basement, where we were sure Supreme would be. Eric and Squanky were standing over Supreme as he worked out on the bench press.

"Supreme, you need to go home. Your family's looking for you," I said.

Supreme continued pressing.

"You got this, Su. Keep pushing," Squanky said.

"No, seriously dude, you need to go home," A. T. said.

"For what? What's going on?" Eric asked.

A. T. opened his mouth. I put my hands on his chest, letting him know it wasn't our place to tell. "There are police cars in front of your house. You need to go," I said.

Supreme struggled to push the bar up onto the bar holder. Squanky grabbed the bar and guided it to the rack. Supreme sat up and smirked, thinking we were pranking him. He searched my face for deception but found only sincerity.

Eric followed him out of the basement, but Supreme turned and stopped him as if he knew it was a family-only situation. Eric nodded, then patted Supreme on the shoulder.

I sat on the empty weight bench and rolled the dumbbells away with my foot. The workout was over. No more weight could be lifted that night.

Days later, I approached the fellas sitting on the stoop. They looked lost. Eric hit me with news that pained worse than any slam: Mr. Griffin had died, slaughtered in the street.

For weeks, the reminder remained on the broken sidewalk where the roots of the oak tree struggled to rise. Only the rain, the same rain that nourished the tree, could wash Mr. Griffin's blood through the cracks.

Discarded.

Party Time

"Traci's having a party?" I asked.

A. T., Alphonso, even Keith seemed to be in the know. Unfazed by my non-invitation, I knew what had to be done.

Later that day, Alfie, A. T., and Kenny were leaning against Joe McKinney's Nova while I stood in the middle of the street, all of us taking turns gulping the fine $1.99 wine. We scoped out the dudes and dudettes going into Traci's backyard. With enough Mad Dog 20/20 soaking into my chest, I stashed the bottle in my jacket pocket. I was ready to crash the party.

From the backyard, I descended through the cellar doors behind Alphonso and Kenny as A. T. brought up the rear. I ducked to avoid smacking my head on the low ceiling of the dank basement.

Sweet chickadees doused in sweat came into focus as my eyes adjusted to the scant swirling light from the disco ball. Mantronix's "Fresh Is the Word" pummeled the walls, and the bass thumped through the speakers. I pulled the Mad Dog from my coat pocket and took a swig.

"Is that Mantronix or Ultra Magnetic?" I asked A.T.

"What?" he said.

The 808 kick drum made talking useless. I twisted my way through the heap of clammy bodies looking for a dry spot to sip and chill. My winding paused when I found myself chest to chest with *her*. I didn't know who she was, but she was *it*. Balls of light crossed her face long enough for me to glimpse the luster of her eyes. Caught in the party's web, our bodies mashed together, involuntarily at first, but MC Shan, KRS-One, and Kool Moe Dee kept us connected. Swaying and sweating, dancing and grinding.

The Mad Dog said, *Grab her waist and pull her closer.* I obeyed. She slid her arms through mine, stimulating my manhood, which I pressed into her. Then we kissed. And kept kissing. The fellas were watching. Females were watching. The watching heightened the experience. I heard a female—maybe Renita?—say, "Humph."

I swooned in the approval or disapproval. Mad Dog said, *To hell with them; keep kissing.* So I did. *Who is she?* I needed to find out. I pulled my tongue out of her mouth and said, "Let's go outside."

I clutched her hand and guided her through the frenzy, then through the backyard and across the street. The chilly night air evaporated my sweat. The streetlamps highlighted the Nova. I turned as she stepped into the illumination. All her facial features—her eyes, nose, teeth—were bigger than I remembered.

Good-gotta-mighty! I tried to position myself at an angle more beneficial to her and myself. Nothing worked. Before any of the fellas came to look, I said, "Let's go back downstairs." We walked through the backyard. Before I descended into the basement, I pulled the Mad Dog from my pocket and chucked it into the garbage can.

Discarded.

The Fall(s)

Before it became "Dead End," it was simply "the Shortcut" since it provided a quick route from North Seventh to Haledon Avenue. We changed the name to "the Pit" because it sounded harder, more menacing. We were kidding ourselves.

The fellas enjoyed laughter way too much and violence way much less. Harm came mostly from the lighthearted wisecracking that merely bruised ego or punctured esteem. Whereas other cliques considered outsiders a threat, we welcomed them.

My cousin Tootsie, Rocky's youngest brother, rarely visited the Pit. If I wanted to see him, I had to go to North Fourth Street, a block in heavy rotation on police scanners. Tootsie wore the Cazals and fat-laced Adidas with the matching sweatsuit, like all the die-hard fans of Run-DMC. His only deviation from their appearance was his curly kit. It was clear who he wanted to be, and wannabees were easy targets.

"You big fake Michael Jackson. You big broke-ass Billy Dee Williams. You big Sugar-less Ray Leonard–looking…."

Someone must've cracked on Tootsie's curly kit or his Run-DMC-ish appearance. Whatever the reason, our lighthearted snaps didn't roll off his back like the Jerry curl juice did. I noticed his withdrawal from our gabfest. His lower lip rested on his knuckles.

He was contemplating his next chess move, or perhaps his next activator purchase; I couldn't be certain.

Tootsie leaped to his feet, saying, "I'll be back." He bopped off, leaving behind a trail of snickers from the fellas and a concerned look from me. My intuition urged me to convince the fellas to take a walk, but they wanted to keep yukking it up.

We stood up when we saw them charging up the landing. The gang's swagger was familiar. It said they were ready to rumble. Tootsie led Damion, Booty, Foster, and big Joe Parks.

Joe Parks was solid and built to trample opposition, so much that he was the running back of Kennedy's football team. Normally, when shit was about to go down and family arrived, they brought a sense of security—not this time.

"Now talk that shit," Tootsie said.

Tootsie's eyes darted from person to person, searching for, hoping for, a response from anyone. He got nothing unless confused looks counted.

"Who's tough now?" he said.

What shit was he talking about? Anthony sat on the rail while Eric, Alfie, and I stood with our backs pinned to the wall. Without a specific target, the crew's hostility stalled. Then Kenny strolled up; his timing couldn't have been more tragic.

"Whaddup," he said.

His "whaddup" was a mixture of curiosity and courtesy. But in that powder keg—which Kenny had wandered into with a match—it meant *What do you want to do?* Either it was an extreme misinterpretation or downright ignorance; either way, the "whaddup" turned into a battle cry.

"What the hell you say?" Joe spoke out of the side of his mouth as if he had a hook in it. Kenny raised his eyebrows while searching for the right response.

"I wasn't talking to you," Kenny said.

"I know you wasn't talking to me, or you'd get fucked up," Joe said.

"I'm outta here. I'm going home," Kenny said. He started the thirty-yard journey home.

"Oh, you going to get something!" Joe huffed before tearing after him.

Kenny broke out in his wobbly run. Joe barreled down on him, then cold-cocked Kenny with a blow to the back of his head. Kenny reeled forward and stumbled into a fence. Joe planted his feet and slugged him in the ribs, dropping Kenny to his knees. Everyone rushed toward the assault. Kenny curled into a ball, protecting his vital organs, while Joe kept pounding.

Tootsie and his crew charged behind, amped up, ready to *get some*. They shouted, "Who else want some?" Back to back, they bounced, fists balled, warding off anyone who dared to step in. Joe backed away with a blank expression from Kenny's motionless body.

"Let's get out of here," Joe said. He ran toward Haledon Avenue with the rest of the sons of bitches. Kenny lay on the ground as the fellas gazed down, dazed.

"Ohhhhh lawwwwd nooo!"

It was a cry filled with the pain that only a mother can feel. The type of wail a mom makes when she sees her son lying on the ground unconscious and uncertain if he's alive. Ms. Queenie ran out of her slippers, dropped to her knees, and cradled Kenny.

"Call 911! Call 911!" she screamed.

Ms. Queenie rocked her son in her arms until the paramedics pulled him out of her grip. Kenny left the pit on a gurney. His mom's wailing punctured the cavity where my heart was supposed to have been.

"What happened?" The question was repeated as tenant after tenant opened their doors. I couldn't stay in the pit any longer. I started walking, confused. What had happened? Everything had happened—anger had happened; fear had happened; life had happened; terrible shit had happened.

Questions tormented me. Why hadn't they helped Kenny? Why hadn't we helped Kenny? Why hadn't I helped Kenny? Did I have more loyalty to my cousin or my homeboy? We were cowards. I was a coward. The long walk ended with me standing in the middle of the narrow footbridge that hovered over the Great Falls. The cascade was a titan hurling tons of water into the pit below, from which a mist rose and sprinkled my face. I stayed on the bridge as long as I could.

Discarded.

Defender

Tiffany stroked my bare chest after our second round of "doing it." *This is what the hoopla was all about*, I thought. I don't remember how or when we started our thing; I only remember the glorious outcomes. I lay in her bed this time thinking, *You Jane. Me Tarzan.* Then Tiffany rose and went into the bathroom, and I noticed her love handles. I thought, *You big, big Jane. Me Tarzan*, and chuckled under my breath.

Is that a hair? A lonely follicle had sprouted from the center of my chest. Hopefully, it was the first of many to come. My thoughts rambled until one made me sit up: *What if someone comes home?* I sprang from her bed and fumbled around the room, looking for my tighty-whities, which Tiffany dangled until I noticed. I slipped into my Nike sweatsuit, then laced up one of my kicks. Tiffany handed me my other sneaker and watched me with a maternal gaze. She didn't want me to leave, but I didn't cave.

Besides, it wasn't safe for me to lie around when, at any second, her eldest brother might pop up. Maurice supposedly preferred young boys. And although I wasn't as young as the ones he supposedly wanted, I wasn't willing to put my ass on the line, betting he could resist it.

I glided along North Fifth Street, smelling myself. *Ahh, the smell of fresh sex. Is this what everyone's been doing? Who should I ask? Who could I ask?* No one. It wasn't something I could brag about due to the rumors about Tiffany's easiness. At least Maurice had preferences; supposedly, Tiffany didn't.

One snow day, I invited Tiffany to come over; I was planning to use my weight bench for something it wasn't designed for. I led the way down the icy stairs and turned in time to see her slip and bust her butt. I shouldn't have laughed, but I did. Way too hard. Apparently, that was the only emotion I had ever expressed to her— her words, not mine. After my experience with Mietta, my guard was up. I wasn't hardened, but I was less of a gentleman. Because of that, Tiffany eventually found someone else to "do it" to. She caught herself a Kennedy knight in shining football armor.

By junior year all my classes bored me, except history. Cutting individual classes meant facing Mr. Sherman, so it was easier to skip the whole day. Playing hooky alone was a drag, so I picked up the phone and dialed a number that at that point was a hit or miss. My dangalang shifted in my drawers when Tiffany answered.

"Whatcha doing?" I asked.

"Going to school. What else?" Tiffany said.

"You want to come over?"

She did. I waited at the door, eager to do what we'd done in the past. After we did what we did, she left without being prompted, which struck me as being both odd and fortuitous. I clicked on the TV and lay in the bed watching it. The phone rang. I didn't answer it because no one should've been home. Ms. Smith, our sixtysomething neighbor, was known to rat me out. The phone rang again. Damn. It had to be Tiffany. Maybe she'd left something. Her voice trembled, which I mistook for excitement, thinking maybe she wanted another round. I lay back against the headboard, thinking, *Spit it out.*

"Joe is mad," Tiffany said.

I sat up. "What? Why he mad?"

"'Cause he knew I was with you."

"How the hell could he know that?"

"'Cause I told him."

You told Joe. The running back. The dude who runs over mafuckers for a living. The monster who pummeled my boy Kenny into unconsciousness, who by the grace of God didn't die or have any recollection of the assault. You told that Joe that we had sex? Have you ever heard of a lie? Why in the world would you tell that maniac you were at my house? I wanted to scream all that into the receiver, but I held it together.

"Why would you tell him that?" I said calmly.

"Because he was here when you called."

Every iota of my attention went to the earpiece of the phone. As if staring at it would lead me out of my profound confusion. I buried my face in the palm of my hand, shaking my head in disbelief.

"So you left your boyfriend at your house in order to come to mine?"

"I didn't know he was going to be waiting here for me when I got back," she said.

I slammed the phone onto the receiver, trying to break it. I paced around the apartment, coming to terms with my fate. My run with life was coming to an end. I would never know what it would feel like to graduate. To have kids. To ride a pony. My poor mother and sister. Tasha would finally get her own room.

The next day at school, I avoided the popular hallways and bathrooms. I took back stairwells. Peeked around corners. And arrived at all my classes at the last second.

Joe had a reputation for sucker-punching, and if I wasn't careful, things could suddenly go dark and I'd wake up with cracked ribs, no teeth, and no recollection.

I maintained consciousness the entire day. And the next. By week's end, I'd started to feel as if longevity was in my future and let my guard down. Maybe as a man, Joe knew it wasn't my fault, or perhaps he realized there was nothing to be gained from mucking me up. For all the uncertainty, there was one thing I was certain about: I would never know his reasoning because I damn sure wasn't going to ask.

On Wednesday the following week, I peeled a Boogie Down Productions flyer off a telephone pole, intending to show the fellas. I was certain they would want to attend. The club's downtown location meant it was within walking distance, so no cab hopping would be necessary. The weekend was going to be phenomenal.

On Thursday, I skipped school. Again.

On Friday, on my way to gym class, I stopped at the water fountain inside the industrial arts class. The ice-cold water hit the back of my throat, and a little ran down my cheek and snaked down inside my collar. I wiped my lips and turned to see Joe Parks.

"You come to school yesterday?" he asked. It was odd that he was taking an interest in my schedule, but I didn't think much of it.

"Nah," I said, then turned my back to him and walked to gym class.

On Friday night after the concert, my boys, who had been extremely rowdy a few blocks earlier, had grown quiet. I stopped at the top of the dark hill. Blab, Messiah's yes man and our new homey, stood in front of Supreme. Behind Supreme stood a teary-eyed Messiah. An ugly cry was imminent.

"What's wrong with Messiah?" I asked.

"You just said 'his father,'" Blab said.

Never would I have made the same mistake Jaima had made. I knew Messiah's father had recently died of AIDS. Messiah's balled-up fists meant an apology wasn't going to be enough.

"Oh shit," I said.

Let me explain how I got here.

That night, a half-hour earlier, Messiah, A. T., Supreme, and I were on our way home from the Cheetah Lounge. Boogie Down Productions had performed their newly released song, "The South Bronx." I was sporting a new leather jacket, and in the words of Dougie Fresh, I was "fresh to death like a million bucks."

The concert ended without a brawl, and that was reason enough to celebrate. I continued to party, doing the Wop as I walked ahead of the fellas. I bobbed my head from side to side until I got pinged in the back of it with a penny. Somebody was disrespecting my dance moves.

"Quit playing," I said. "People hate to see a brother having a good time."

Everyone laughed. We continued up Temple Street. A few yards later, another penny bounced off my noggin.

"Whoever did it, their mother," I said. A few steps later, the ping of another penny.

"Your mother two times," I said.

"Say 'Whoever did it, their father,'" A. T. said.

"Whoever did it, their father," I said.

We continued past the rec center, past the CCP projects, onto Circle Avenue, past the firehouse, and up toward Clinton Hill until we landed on North Fourth street. Where I turned around.

And that's how I got here.

North Fourth Street transformed before my eyes. The parked cars became ropes; the blacktop became a mat; my boys became referees. The bell was about to ring. All that was missing was the ring announcer.

"In this corner, the challenger from the Pit, a very, very concerned Rodney Laney."

The people in the crowd shake their heads pitifully.

"In this corner, we have the reigning champion, snot-nosed crying Messiah."

"Messiah, I didn't know you were the one to hit me. Otherwise, I wouldn't have said it," I said.

"I know you didn't know, but..." Messiah said. His eyes locked in on A. T. "But he knew."

"In this corner, the guy with a cheap smile who just realized he's in deep shit, A. T."

"And that's why he said to say 'his father,'" Messiah continued.

I gladly accepted my role as a referee.

"A. T., why you say 'Say his father?'" I asked.

"Man, I was just playin'. I ain't know you was gonna say it."

"Why you say to say my father in the first place?" Messiah said.

Messiah's breath quickened. He had to do something to stop the tears; breaking a jaw would probably do the trick. He took off his hoodie and threw up his hands.

"You knew what you were doing," Messiah said. A. T. didn't remove his jacket. There wasn't enough time.

"Man, go 'head with dat," A. T. said.

"Put your hands up," Messiah demanded.

Messiah began closing the distance. A. T. stepped back with his hands still at his side.

"You better put your hands up," Messiah said. That was Messiah's final warning before throwing his infamous Bolo punch. And then, similar to the Frank/Jaima scuffle, something inexplicable happened.

A. T. ducked, so low his back pockets scraped the ground, but when he sprang back up, he was a car's length away from Messiah and facing the opposite direction. He'd pulled off a *Matrix* move— before there was a *Matrix*. It was a reverse moonwalk duck. It was a move that would've impressed the real Messiah. Supreme and I looked at each other, trying to make sense of what we'd witnessed.

"How the hell did he do that?" we asked.

We erupted in laughter, and as much as he didn't want to, Messiah cracked up too. We clowned the hell out of A. T. Of course, he didn't think it was that funny. Instead of Wopping, I started doing the A. T. shuffle. We didn't stop busting on A. T. until we reached Roger's.

The warning bells hanging over the grimy glass door jangled as I entered Roger's. I noticed that Defender, my game, was available. I dropped two dollars on the counter in exchange for quarters. Barbara stood waiting in her bulldoggish way until I realized my mistake. I collected the singles off the counter, then placed them into her palm. The community's matriarch had rules and shit. Thanks to her rules, the store was a safe haven. Everyone knew to leave the bullshit at the door. Those warning bells swung both ways.

It had taken me a long time to get good at Defender due to its complexity. After dropping dozens of quarters and getting blown up over and over again, I'd finally gotten good enough to put my name in the game.

The fellas hung outside while I made a poor man's Mount Rushmore with four quarters on the panel, letting everyone know I planned on playing hero for as long as my coins permitted.

Holding the joystick tight, I thrust my ship with tight maneuvers, firing missile after missile, blowing up aliens, protecting humanity from the evil mutants, saving the day, and preventing my world from annihilation. Defender's hyperspace button was best used in critical situations only, when death was imminent, because once you went into hyperspace, you disintegrated, then reintegrated into another point in space that could be better, or worse, or sometimes you would explode for no reason. I blasted away until A. T. appeared at my shoulder.

"Yo, Rodney! Why Joe Parks wanna fight you?" he asked.

I scoffed, figuring it was a weak attempt at payback for the earlier ridicule.

"Yeah, right," I said.

"I'm serious. He's outside telling everyone he's gonna fuck you up."

It didn't make sense. Why would he want to fight me? I hadn't done anything to him. *Lately.* I resumed focus on saving the world. A. T. left, defeated again.

The clank of the warning bells made the hairs on my neck rise and called attention to whoever or whatever it was that stood behind me.

"Yo, Rodney, I'm going to fuck you up," I heard.

Over my shoulder, I glimpsed at a real mutant standing in the aisle, blocking the door. The bells jangled again and again and again as people came in to see. If only I could go into hyperspace mode for real.

Barbara placed her Louisville Slugger on the counter, a reminder of the store's policy. The store cleared out. Joe's reputation for sucker-punching opponents wasn't lost on me, but I kept playing with him at my back. I couldn't let him see me sweat, or hear my heartbeat, or…see me sweat. He lunged toward me as if he was going to break the store's rules, but thank God, Messiah stepped in between us. Barbara picked up the bat.

"Take it outside," she warned.

"You gotta come outside, Rodney," Joe said.

The bells clanged. One after the other, my ships were blown to smithereens. I'd been stunted. I stalled as long as my quarters allowed while thinking of a way to escape.

The last George Washington stared at me as if he knew I was prolonging the unpreventable. I frisked myself for more coins, turning my pockets inside out like the guy on the bankruptcy card in Monopoly.

This store sucks for having only one way out, I thought. While I was eyeing the storage closet, Barbara was eyeing me. I wanted to ask to borrow her Slugger. She escorted me to the door with a nod. Options blazed through my mind while I bit my lip. *Do I roll up my sleeves? These sleeves are brand new. That's it.*

My new leather blazer would be my excuse. Everyone would understand that I didn't want to ruin my new gear. I hoped. I was faster than Kenny, and I had the element of surprise. *What's the worst that could happen? I get clowned—the way we clowned A. T.?* He'd created a brand-new way to duck, so he couldn't say shit. Hell, it would be something we could all laugh at later. It was settled.

I knelt down and tied my laces tight. I could feel Barbara's stare but couldn't face her. I eased open the door, preventing the bells from tattling, then stepped into the doorway. *Aww, shit!*

Who'd done the promotion for this, Don King? The mob was spread as wide as I could register in a glance.

"There he is," someone said.

"You ready to take this ass whooping, Rodney?" Joe said. His remark roused the crowd.

The path to 113 Haledon Avenue was clear. I could be in my living room in ninety seconds flat. I looked to Messiah and said, "Hold my jacket."

The adrenaline abolished all but one thought: *Don't let him grab me.* My knuckles guarded my chin; fear guided my focus. Joe rushed forward, throwing two quick hooks, hoping to decapitate me. I parried and stepped to my left, guided by gut instinct. I was still conscious—a good thing. Each miss counted as a victory. I settled into the fight, and each time he threw a punch, I reacted with a visceral counterattack, guided by the one thought: *Don't let him grab me.*

Tunnel vision shrunk my reality down to Joe's fists and dark eyes. Between each breath, *Don't let him grab me.* Then a lone voice from the crowd said, "Rodney's fucking him up."

That voice broke my concentration and widened my scope, revealing Joe's lacerated forehead, bruised eyes, and trickles of blood beneath his nose. And that's when another thought came to mind. *I can knock him out.*

I started with plan B. Instead of being on the heels of my Pumas, I raised myself up on my toes and moved forward, searching for the sweet spot on his chin to send him night-night.

I should've stuck with plan A. I threw an overzealous right hook that threw me off balance, landing me where I'd promised myself I wouldn't be: in deep shit and within Joe's grasp.

I struggled to free myself from his steel clutch. Then he tried to go low, but I kept my footing by kicking my legs back to lower my center of gravity, remembering that's how Crab and Mark had gotten me. Then he tried to sweep my legs, but I wasn't falling for that either. The grappling carried us from the sidewalk into the street, energizing the crowd while halting traffic. Joe's football stamina kept up his aggression, while fatigue changed the momentum, becoming his ally and my nemesis.

He muscled me against a station wagon, then grabbed the backs of my thighs and drove me onto the hood. The booming thud echoed. I could feel females wince; I wanted to assure them that it sounded harder than it felt. Nevertheless, any chance of victory appeared to be slipping away along with my energy. His viciousness turned savage when he sank his teeth into my shoulder. This big, greasy, puffy-eyed, skinned-up-forehead motherfucker was biting me. Biting was forbidden.

"Only punks bite," I said.

It was a disqualifying move in the hood. I let everyone know: "He's biting me. He's biting me." I could hear snickering and disgraceful moans. Joe heard it too, but he didn't give a damn. "I'm going to need a tetanus shot," I hollered.

In the middle of our brawl, I wondered: *How could anyone be this violent?* His anger baffled me and showed no signs of deescalating, evident by him sticking his fingers in my eyes, a move I'd only seen on *The Three Stooges.* This battle had become a farce. Composed, I asked: "Can someone get him out of my eyes, please?"

We were pushed apart, two boxers in the fifteenth round, gasping for breath. Joe's eye-gouging had displaced my contact lenses. *Great.* They were hiding in the back of my eyeballs. A car honked, wanting to pass through the dogfight. The pause gave me time for my lenses to snap back onto my pupils.

Round two.

If we'd started as two centurions, we ended as two centenarians. The score had been settled as far as I was concerned, but accepting defeat wasn't in Joe's playbook. With a final effort, he lunged forward, collaring me again. We fell backward; Joe landed on top. I knew if he got his jumbo fists free, he would pummel the shit out of me. I locked his arms with mine above his elbows, using all of my remaining might. Two hands snatched Joe by his shoulders, yanking him off me. He stumbled backward, then buckled against a car, finished.

"It ain't over, Rodney. It ain't over," he said.

I took the hand that advanced toward me with a solid grip, feeling my weight lifted as I was heaved to my feet. I regained my footing. After pushing Joe aside and lifting me up, Kenny helped dust me off. The two of us, along with Messiah, headed toward Jefferson Street, away from the crowd, then turned the corner.

The night air-dried the sweat and blood. Messiah handed me my jacket. The pain in my shoulder prevented me from putting it on. I draped it across my hand, which began throbbing. I wanted to ask Kenny why he hadn't taken revenge on the exhausted Joe, but I couldn't.

"What happened?" Mom asked when I walked through the door.

"I had a fight."

Mom kneeled to inspect my hand. Her half-mast eyes passed over the puffiness that wrapped around my pinkie finger and stretched down the back of my hand to my wrist. The swelling had created a meat muffin. She iced my injury to attenuate the swelling, then asked if I thought I needed medical attention. I decided it would be best to go to the emergency room.

When the tetanus shot was administered, I didn't flinch. X-rays showed a hairline fracture in my hand. The nurse wrapped my hand in a wet, gauzy material that would harden into my first cast. She rolled the plaster-like gauze gently around my open hand, around my wrist, and up my forearm, occasionally looking up at me, then eventually broke the silence: "You're done."

I pondered one of the many questions Mom had asked before taking me to the hospital: "Did you win?"

News of the fight spread throughout Kennedy's homerooms and hallways. The day after the fight, Brandon Presley, the guy who'd made a lasting impression when he drilled Wendell in the chest in school twelve and who was also one of Joe's teammates, approached me.

"I heard you beat Joe up?" he asked.

"We had a fight," I said.

Brandon, who had become a huge LL Cool J fan, gave me a fist bump, then walked away looking as if he couldn't live without his radio.

Joe's version of events differed from mine. Some said he claimed the bruises had come from a brawl with his brother. Funny, I felt the same way since I had suffered so many bruises from my "brothers."

Discarded.

The Question

A peculiar expression colored Mom's face as she placed a bowl of chicken soup in front of me. "I'm trying something new," she said. Her expression blended a nurturing pride with a hint of concern, piquing my curiosity. "Bob wants us to be a family. He cherishes you like a son," Mom said.

Did he pop the question? I wondered, *or are there way too many last names on the mailbox?*

"He wants to know if you would consider calling him Dad," Mom said.

I took a long slurp of the savory soup and pondered. I should've seen that coming from an incident at work when I walked into the kitchen while Bob was conversing with a client. The client gave me an approving nod, saying: "He's got a good work ethic. Is this your son?"

"Yes," Bob replied.

I am? I forgot why I'd walked into the kitchen. The notion was duct-taped to my mind. I rationalized that he had to get through the paperwork and the quick answer to the client was convenient.

Back in our own kitchen, Mom said: "What do you think about that?"

I slurped down another tablespoon and wondered if it was the steamy broth or calling Bob Dad that warmed my belly.

Discarded.

The Big Move

Rodney Miller," I said.

I was checking to see how the name rolled off the tongue. Bob had asked Mom once if I would consider changing my last name. Miller? It could be my tagline right before a squabble: "Who talking shit on me? Well, guess what? It's Miller time."

The cheesiness tickled me as I stood in the bathroom wrestling with my tie. I noticed if I tilted my shoulders fifteen degrees, it appeared straight. I untied the knot and tried again, determined to get it right.

Later that day in the church, Uncle Gucci stood in his formal Coast Guard uniform with white gloves, standing next to Dad, who was dressed in a black suit, black tie, and white shirt. At the altar, I stood sporting my new gray three-piece suit with a white carnation. Tasha stood next to Aunt Mildred as Mom, dressed in a flowery crown and handsome white gown, did the wedding two-step down the aisle.

The pastor of Canaan Baptist asked, "Who gives this woman to be married to this man?"

Mom's nervous, vulnerable, and proud look put a lump in my throat. I adjusted my clip-on tie and said, "I do."

Discarded.

My "Movie" Ends

My eyes opened. I took a moment to orient myself, then leaned forward to stretch my back. I checked my Movado. The seemingly forty-five minutes that had passed were really three hours. Careful not to disturb the other meditators, I slipped into my footwear and read the "coexist" vow. The bells barely jangled when I closed the door and walked onto Teaneck Road.

I couldn't take my eyes off the great blue sky. The boldness of the clouds moved me. It was clear why so many spiritual texts referenced the skies as heaven. It was as if it were the first time I could truly see them. I wanted to point them out to people and say, "Can you see the beauty?"

My meditation sessions lasted from one to six hours, depending on my schedule. After a month of discarding, I felt energized and lighter physically and mentally. And the most fascinating aspect was how my reality had become incredibly vivid. With each meditation, the speed at which I could discard increased. I could fast-forward through the first ten years of my life within minutes. I wondered if I'd lose the memories altogether. This was always a concern for people new to the meditation. I was and will always be able to recall the memories, but without the negative emotion that bad memories have attached to them.

"But what about the joy memories bring?" you might ask.

The joy I could now experience in the present was greater than the pleasure that came from a memory.

One memory of them all is the one that broke me.

When I was living on North Fourth street, Eddie and I were sleeping in my bed when I had an accident. Mom discovered the pee and whooped me where I lay, wet drawers and all. It was a stinging memory.

Before meditation, I only had the capacity to view that memory from a perspective formed as a child. During a discard session, I saw the scenario from a superior perspective. It was as if I zoomed out to see the entire picture, which included Mom's aspect. Her frustration with her son resonated with me as I meditated. Being able to see that charged memory from that third-person viewpoint created real empathy. I say real empathy because I was able to feel her emotions while not feeling my own. That bears repeating, but I won't repeat it.

Pause and think about if you've ever done that: looked at a situation where you felt you were wronged, but from the other person's viewpoint, while your emotions have been nullified.

Forgiveness wasn't an issue. I didn't have to forgive Mom; actually, it was the opposite. My selfishness had permitted me to see that and all the following events only from my own perspective. And for that, I owed Mom and the universe an apology.

My personal history had created a story about women that I was unaware of. The powerful realization of that perspective changed me and released profound guilt. It was so overwhelming that my eyes watered, and tears from the understanding flowed.

The Meditation

I was working on an eight-day Alaskan cruise and had just left the buffet with a slice of cake and two scoops of ice cream when I read a sign: "Secrets to a flatter stomach." Hmmm. *I like secrets, and I like flat stomachs,* I thought, but not as much as I like lemon pound cake and butter pecan ice cream. The workshop was starting in ten minutes, enough time for me to finish dessert and make my stomach less flat.

During the seminar, a Yugoslavian-looking dude in a muscle shirt said, "Fat reduction comes in percentages: 20 percent from exercise, 30 percent from nutrition, and 50 percent from detoxification." He continued, saying that the buildup of fat came from toxins from coffee, refined sugars, aspartame, and other chemicals such as phosphorous acid. *I have to give up coffee? I'm outta here.*

All of those chemicals overworked the liver, he said, which eventually made fat cells unusable for energy. At least that's what I think he said; his accent was thicker than his biceps. I kept trying to place the accent. Maybe he was Ukrainian?

He continued telling us how the process depleted metabolism and energy. Once the energy flow is altered, fat begins to get deposited in the lymph node areas, like the stomach, neck, hips, and chin. The Croatian(?) went on to say that the intestines were twenty-four feet long, but only eight feet can be checked out by colonoscopy, and that's why colon cancer has the highest mortality rate of all the cancers in America. (If ever I wanted to google something, it was right then.) He then mentioned how the intestines could hold seven to eight meals. *Not if I drink coffee*, I thought.

I had been meditating for nineteen months and was enlightened to the "true body and true mind," which extend beyond the physical body and psychological mind, so I listened to the presentation with a raised eyebrow. I started thinking, *What difference would it make if I had a flat stomach with a fat head?* A head clogged with toxic chemicals of a different nature.

Then the Serbian(?) started talking about John Wayne, probably because everyone in the seminar was at least seventy years old. He said John Wayne's favorite meal was steak and potatoes. When he died of colon cancer, they found forty-five pounds of undigested meat in his colon. Yuck! My question was, "Why would they even look for that?"

Finally, he came to the solution of detoxing to put the body in an alkaline state, which is the state of homeostasis.

"In the alkaline state, no disease can exist," he said.

Once the body is detoxified, the liver, "the most important organ," begins to function optimally and stops storing the toxins in fat cells, and you'll obtain that elusive flat stomach. The secret to obtaining the alkaline state? Algae pills. All this to sell us bottles of algae. I didn't fact-check any of this because the ship's Wi-Fi was spotty—right when I needed it most.

He put the attainment of a flat stomach in percentages and compared it to building a house. Detoxification represented the foundation and was 50 percent of the process, as I mentioned. The house itself represented nutrition and was 30 percent, while exercise represented the roof, completing the remaining 20 percent.

At the conclusion, he asked if there were any questions. I didn't think he could answer the questions I had. Science can determine the toxic buildup in the body, but can it determine what constitutes a toxic buildup in the mind? What specifically are the pollutants? How do you achieve mind and body homeostasis? I wondered what would happen if we applied this approach to our mind/body/spirit complex. I determined that the foundation for detoxing the mind would be meditation, and the nutrition would be the material we allow to seep into our consciousness.

The year 2020 was one of the most divisive I have experienced. Whenever I observed the blue political party versus the red, it was always in the context best described by a passage in *A Course in Miracles*:

> What perception sees and hears appears to be real because it permits into awareness only what conforms to the wishes of the perceiver. This leads to a world of illusions, a world which needs constant defense precisely because it is not real. When you have been caught in the world of perception you are caught in a dream. You cannot escape without help, because everything your senses show merely witnesses to the reality of the dream.[1]

---

1   Foundation for Inner Peace. 1996. *A Course in Miracles*. Viking Penguin. *"All quotes are from A Course in Miracles, copyright ©1992, 1999, 2007 by the Foundation for Inner Peace, 448 Ignacio Blvd., #306, Novato, CA 94949, acim.org and info@acim.org, used with permission."*

I remember a few years ago, while I was in a class, a young Jewish student talked about her trip to Israel. She was asked about the Gaza conflict and how it had impacted the locals. I found her casual response insightful. She said, "Everyone seemed to get along until they started watching TV."

Technology initially developed to connect us has played an enormous role in dividing the world. The connectivity we have to our cell phones, computers, and televisions puts our minds under an onslaught of pictures. Many are designed to market and entertain, but many are designed to manipulate and coerce us. The worst images create fear and anger and even incite riots.

While I was visiting my son in Colorado Springs, I decided to explore the area. It was easy to meander for hours because of how the suburban division was arranged. It was connected by walkways and bike paths that flowed seamlessly into the next neighborhood. As I continued roaming, I came to a cul-de-sac. A white man came out of his home carrying something underneath his arm that was long and slender. I stopped walking.

The night before this, a video of the shooting of Ahmaud Arbery, an unarmed Black man, by a white man had gone viral and ended up in my inbox. I didn't watch all of the horrific video because I knew where it was headed. And enough was enough.

That video caused pictures to start forming; images of Black men being shot flashed through my mind in milliseconds. And as I walked in Colorado Springs the next day, my internal voice—I call him Jerome—sounded off: *I am a Black man, in an all-white neighborhood, in an unfamiliar city, in an unfamiliar state....*

I stopped walking, not from the emotion the *thought* was trying to generate but from my awareness of the thought's attempt to create fear. I paid attention to my inner Jerome. Then I started a walking meditation and discarded the imagery of the fatal shootings, which prevented that imagery from creating an unreal fear in my present moment. According to my meditation, we are continually projecting our past experiences onto reality, and therefore not living in the real world.

An article from the *Harvard Gazette*'s Health and Medicine section entitled "The Power of Picturing Thoughts" conveys an idea similar to what I was experiencing:

> Your mind can produce all images that were stored in the past. When your eyes are closed light can not enter through them. However, your brain can produce enough light internally and projects the images you have already stored to a screen that you can see in your mind.[2]

It's the accumulation and repetition of these electronic images that begin to dictate how our lives unfold. It's clear how this can be not only limiting but, in extreme cases, even deadly.

What would happen if we all looked at the images in our minds and eliminated their ability to control us by triggering our fears, anger, or hatred? Would the mindless violence end? Would we be able to see the real world and not the illusory world we've created from memories? Only you can find out how your pictures affect you. And until you do a thorough inward-focused self-examination, you will remain clueless as to their impact.

---

2   Reuell, Peter, "The Power of Picturing Thoughts," *Harvard Gazette*, May 11, 2017, https//news.harvard.edu/gazette/story/2017/05/visual-images-often-intrude-on-verbal-thinking-study-says/aei.

Of course, we can't avoid images. Many times images are necessary to galvanize people to take action. We've all been impacted by the murder of George Floyd. And for anyone who has seen the video, the mere mention of it will bring up the image. And along with the image will come an emotion. What emotion do you feel as you think about the video?

Is it contempt, anger, sadness, indifference, or fear? Did you assign blame? If so, who was to blame? Now ask yourself where the emotion came from. Was it from the author's words or the reader's memory?

If you pondered those questions even for a second, your mental projector started and began projecting your habitual imagery into the film in your head. Because only you can see that film, it's an illusion. It's your mind movie. (All you need now is popcorn.)

After my inner Jerome was silenced that day in Colorado Springs, I continued walking, observing the clear blue sky with a mountainous backdrop. Other thoughts formed, arousing my curiosity. I wondered how the world would be different if everyone had the ability to free themselves from their habitual way of thinking. I wondered if we could eradicate the fear that causes violence. I wondered if Trayvon Martin would still be alive as I walked to the home of my son, Trevaughn.

HOW DO WE HEAL?

I went out to promote the meditation center one day. Being on the street reminded me of my early comedy days when I hawked comedy tickets in Times Square for stage time. I approached a gentleman, offering him a meditation pamphlet similar to the one that had gotten me started.

He said, "No, thank you. I pray," and kept walking.

I said, "You know, you can do both."

He paused for a second and said, "You're right," and kept walking.

I have found that devout churchgoers are resistant to meditation. I speculate that it's either because of misunderstandings about meditation or because it's not emphasized in the church as much as prayer. The Bible mentions meditation numerous times. It has been referenced in the book of Psalms nineteen times, often stated as "obedience in the next breath."

Once I asked Mom if she was interested in meditating, and she looked at me as if I was trying to take her Jesus away.

"I'm not trying to take away your wine and crackers, Mom," I said. *I'm just trying to give you some cheese to go with them.*

Meditation and prayer are like peanut butter and jelly, syrup and pancakes, sugar and diabetes—wait, disregard that last analogy, but you get my point.

They are both used in the search for a deeper level of peace, and both can be used during challenging times. There are differences between the two. Prayer is speaking and seeking, while meditation is listening and accepting. Prayer is outward and dependent upon faith, while meditation is inward and doesn't require a belief. Prayer is dualistic, while meditation is oneness. Prayer is time-dependent, meaning it references the future, while meditation resides outside of time and is more concerned with the here and now. Meditation allows for the presence of a divine entity without a philosophy around it, and in that way, it's more inclusive.

The confusion about meditation might start with its original translation. When many people think of meditation, they take the definition as the act of engaging in contemplation or reflection. Many believe it's about focus and concentration. The word "meditation" derives from the Sanskrit word *dhyāna* or *jhāna*, which means "higher contemplation." It can also be translated as "training of the mind" so that one becomes aware and withdraws from the habitual reactions from external stimuli, which ultimately leads to perfect equanimity and enlightenment.

Meditation is not only mentioned in the Bible but in all of the most sacred scriptures of Buddhism, Hinduism, Judaism, and Islam. I haven't read the Koran, but I have watched videos of people who have—because I am a thorough researcher. When asked about meditation, Shabir Ally, president of the Islamic Information and Dawah Centre International, said: "When Muslims perform the absolutions at home at the end of the day, one may want to recollect one's events or one's actions and sort the good from the bad, and ask God to forgive us for what one had done wrong."[3] In essence, meditation is repentance.

Similarly, when one discards pictures, it is also a repentance because to repent means to change one's mind. In order to change your mind, you have to be willing to examine it. Socrates is credited with saying, "The unexamined life is really not worth living." I wouldn't go that far; Socrates sounded a little morbid. I will say that self-examination makes you less of yourself or selfless, and living for others creates a life worth living.

REFLECTIVE MEDITATION

According to the book *Be As You Are: The Teachings of Sri Ramana Maharshi* (who is one of India's most revered spiritual masters): "If you are vigilant and make a stern effort to reject every thought when

---

3   "Q&A: Practicing Meditation in Islam – Dr. Shabir Ally," YouTube video, 6:22 "Let the Quran Speak" 2014 https://youtu.be/atMeDOVrWFs.

it rises you will soon find that you are going deeper and deeper into your own inner self."[4]

Sri Ramana Maharshi continues to say that once you reach a certain level, it is not necessary to make an effort to reject thoughts.

Over time, the release of the pictures taken by my "body cam" freed me from the psychological fears that came with my story: the fear of rejection, failure, and punishment. All those fears were anchored by the emotions attached to them. It's no wonder they call it "baggage." All that excess weight causes tension in the neck, shoulders, and back, like a ninety-pound duffel bag. Carrying that baggage is toxic and keeps you stuck in your habitual way of being.

When you meditate deeply and experience stillness, it's the stillness that watches the thoughts, the judgments, and the motives that pass through your mind. It's the stillness that watches the film that you call your life. In that awareness, you can watch it without the emotional charge, as the silent witness in total awareness. The distance between the thoughts and the witness gives you the ability to respond as opposed to reacting. To meditate is to understand the makeup of your nature and spirit. And you come to know the emptiness that allows consciousness to flourish.

HOW TO DO IT

This meditation is unique, innovative, and counterintuitive. The method is different from mindfulness and breath-focused meditations, but the end result—freedom from suffering—is the same. Whereas many meditations treat thoughts as something to avoid, reflective meditation, in my opinion, embraces them.

---

4   Godman, David.1985. *Be As You Are The Teachings of Sri Ramana Maharshi.*
     :New Delhi:Akash Press.

The requirement to recall the day's events invited thinking and mental activity for me. For example, if I had an argument or was offended by someone, I would replay my day as if it were a film and eliminate the frames one by one. This severed the emotional link to the memory, thereby disempowering it and any story I had created around the incident.

This is why the meditation is a repentance—because it is, in essence, forgiveness. Many meditators have testified that this has helped in their work environment. The act of eliminating all of the amassed pictures of coworkers, supervisors, and bosses lightens the internal burden many people carry home from work.

The tone of this book has been quite humorous—if I say so myself—but here's where the tone changes and things get real or surreal. I'll ask you to suspend judgment and opinions and remain open. I recommend going to a meditation center or going to my website, RodneyLaney.com, for frequently asked questions.

Find a comfortable seated position. For this meditation, no particular body position is required. Sitting up straight will help prevent you from falling asleep. Avoid chairs that are too comfy, as they will put you to sleep faster than a PowerPoint presentation. If you fall asleep easily, you can do this meditation with your eyes open.

Create a state of grace. Choose whatever makes you feel grateful. Let's begin.

Review your day.

Start from the time you awoke. Recall going to the bathroom, getting dressed, checking your phone. Recall your breakfast, chatting with a loved one, and going to work or school. As these pictures and images come into your mind, see them as pictures, Polaroids, or frames in a movie reel that you can freeze. In your mind's eye, burn the pictures. See the images set aflame and burned to a crisp. See the ashes burn and completely disappear. With each frame continue burning. As you move through your day, visualize all your memories this way and burn them all. It might be easy to burn a supervisor or boss, but more difficult to burn a loved one, but remember it's only an image. Feel the relief as each image goes up in flames.

Work your way to the present. Burn the image of yourself as well, sitting where you are. Remember, it's only an image. See all your worries and preoccupations disintegrating. If any of the images persist, keep burning them until they no longer remain. It may be necessary to go through several rounds, especially if you've had a trying day.

Imagine yourself completely free from those images. Keep your mind empty.

Whenever a new image appears, burn it instantly. No thought or image can withstand the 3,000-degree flame you cast it into.

Once you've become accustomed to the daily review, start reviewing your life in its entirety. Start with your earliest childhood memory. Review your life in ten-year increments. Go through as much of your life as time permits. Once you've finished the first ten years, continue on to the next decade, eleven years of age until twenty, then twenty-one to thirty, and so on.

The more you review and discard memories, the more latent memories will begin to arise. These older memories are easy to dwell in. Don't get stuck in them (or else you might end up writing a book!). Burn them up.

Initially, it will take longer to cycle through ten years, but you'll get faster. Eventually, you'll be able to power through a decade of life in under five minutes. The memories won't linger.

Once you've become accustomed to reviewing your entire life, the next step is breaking it down into categories. This is particularly helpful if you find a certain aspect of your life challenging. For example, you can reflect on money, fame, fortune, love, family, work, school, religion, sex, and the future. I caution you to become adept at eliminating images before going into these categories, as they will pull you into a vortex of thought and judgments. Be aware that the most seductive category for men, I'm told, is money, and for women is family.

After a few months, you'll notice you're zipping through your life lived, and you'll start to carry this process into your daily life. You won't even wait until meditation before you start burning up images. You'll burn them up while walking.

When I started discarding the "life lived," I was aggressive and meditated for two to four hours a day—like I said, it was a slow summer. I encourage you to start with twenty minutes and work up to an hour and continue to your soul's content.

This is the first step on the path to a lighter, or "enlightened," you. It is powerful, provocative, and extremely beneficial to most. The results will match your eagerness. Be patient and trust the process, and you'll see how your energy will attract new circumstances that will encourage you to continue your spiritual development. I've said it before, and I'll say it again: Consider going to a center for guided meditation. Building your metaphysical home on the foundation laid by others is sound practice.

BONUS: THE COOL-DOWN

After you've done a round of discarding and feel cleansed, bring your attention to your breath. Feel the inhalation and the exhalation. Focus on your nostrils. Observe the natural flow of your respiration, and allow your breath to flow naturally and unaltered. From this point, any thought that enters into your awareness only needs to be observed and treated as an impersonal object. After you feel you're in a state of focused awareness, move your attention to your body.

Imagine your attention as a small flashlight, and shine it on every part of your anatomy. Start with your toes. Move through each one, then to the balls of your feet, to your instep, then to your heels. You should feel a sensation on each part of the body you bring your attention to. If not, don't worry. Simply allow the sensations to happen naturally. Remember to remain on each body part for only a few seconds.

Bring attention to your calves and continue incrementally moving your attention up. Keep ascending toward your knees, thighs, groin, hips, abdomen, back, chest, shoulders, and down your arms to your hands. Then move up to your neck, chin, lips, cheeks, nose, eyes, and forehead until you reach the tip of your head. Feel the aliveness of the body.

Whenever you feel your thoughts hijacking your meditation, just observe them without judgment, and they will eventually fade. If there are times you feel overwhelmed by thoughts, bring your attention back to your breathing.

Do this meditation daily, preferably in the evening. This simple practice, if done consistently, will yield remarkable results. As your consciousness rises, so will your ability to maintain awareness and focus.

It takes diligence to break free from our programming, and I'm not talking about Netflix. (Although replacing an hour of television with an hour of meditation would be a good thing. You ever wonder why they call it programming? It is hidden in plain sight.)

As with so many new endeavors, we often need assistance for clarity and motivation. If you find yourself unable to do this simple meditation or find your diligence declining, you can obtain assistance by reaching out to my website, RodneyLaney.com.

Once you're freed from yourself, amazing grace awaits. The meditation gave me the inspiration and focus to write this book, an unexpected fringe benefit that set my life on a new trajectory. I am offering you the same profound benefits.

Epilogue

Besides curse words, there were other words Mom prohibited my sister and me from saying. If I said someone was lying, I might've ended up lying on the floor. Instead of using the word "lie," I had to say "telling a story." That term is befitting to what I, and most of us, have been doing: telling ourselves a story.

That's not to say all our life experiences are not valid, or our recall isn't sound. Of course, life offers valuable insights that can enhance our lives, but we don't usually create detrimental narratives around those insights.

It's the events we deem harmful or dangerous that we create a story around, not understanding that those stored images skew our perception in our present-moment reality, particularly when a present situation appears similar to a previous one. And the stronger the initial emotional response, the higher the distortion of the truth.

For those who are afraid to give up their story, just turn to the opening statement in *A Course in Miracles*: "Nothing real can be threatened. Nothing unreal exists."

I love my mom dearly, and our relationship couldn't have been better. And until meditation, I never fully understood her plight because I looked at life only from the perspective of a self-centered person; for that, I apologize. I know that she and all the moms have done their best.

Mom gave me a book titled *A Book of Prayer: 365 Prayers for Victorious Living,* by Stormie Omartian. Here's one of my favorite passages:

> Lord, I pray that You would set me free from my past. Wherever I have made my past my home. I pray that You would deliver me, heal me. And redeem me from it. Help me to let go of anything I have held onto of my past that has kept me from moving into all you have for me. Enable me to put off all the former ways of thinking and feeling and remembering (Ephesians 4:22-24). Give me the mind of Christ so I will be able to understand when I am being controlled by memories of past events. I release my past to You and everyone associated with it so you can restore what has been lost.

Thanks to meditation, I am freed from the ultimate authority—the authority of my story.

I thank you, the reader, for giving me your most precious commodity: your attention.

Acknowledgments

Thanks to Raia King for her encouragement, Geoffery Berwind for his inspiration, and Debra Englander for her optimism. Thanks to my soulmate, my hero, and most beloved fan: my Mom.

About the Author

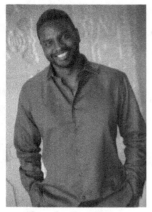

Photo by Natalie Post

Rodney Laney is a veteran of stand-up comedy and the Air Force. His hometown, Paterson, New Jersey inspired the comedy which has led to Laney's numerous television appearances, including *The Late Late Show*, Comedy Central, and HBO. Laney discovered an innovative meditation in 2013 that he wants to share with the world.